Master *your* METaBOLISM

THE ALL-NATURAL (*all-herbal*) WAY TO LOSE WEIGHT

Master *your* METaBOLISM

THE ALL-NATURAL (*all-herbal*) WAY TO LOSE WEIGHT

LEWIS HARRISON

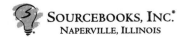

SOURCEBOOKS, INC.
NAPERVILLE, ILLINOIS

Published by Sourcebooks, Inc.
P.O. Box 4410, Naperville, Illinois 60567-4410
(630) 961-3900
FAX: (630) 961-2168
www.sourcebooks.com

Library of Congress Cataloging-in-Publication Data

Harrison, Lewis.
  Master your metabolism : the all-natural (all-herbal) way to lose weight / by Lewis Harrison.
       p. cm.
  Includes bibliographical references and index.
  ISBN 1-4022-0056-0 (pbk. : alk. paper)
  1. Weight loss. 2. Herbs—Therapeutic use. I. Title.
RM222.2 .H2539 2003
613.2'5—dc21

                              2002153632

     Printed and bound in the United States of America
        BG   10 9 8 7 6 5 4 3 2 1

Dedicated to my wife and my hero, Lilia Harrison

Acknowledgments

Thanks to the late Dr. John Christopher, my first herb teacher. Thanks to Jill Hendrickson and Corey Rodin for helping to organize research into the chapter structure. Thanks also to Elizabeth Menendez, Erik Oliva, and especially to Armond Rulhman for the final proofreading and correcting of the manuscript. Special thanks to Noah Lukeman, my agent, for having faith in the value of the book. Thanks to my mother for supporting my writing as a teenager; my natural healing teacher Vincent Collura, who taught me to look at the individual, not the symptoms; and to my spiritual teacher, Huzur Charan Singh Ji, whose wisdom has made my life as smooth as one might ask for.

Table of Contents

Author to Reader

As a long-time teacher, writer, and consultant on health matters, I have often been asked by readers, students, clients, physicians, and practitioners of various healing arts to compile a book about using herbs and spices to facilitate weight loss. Welcome to *Master Your Metabolism*.

You are beginning an exciting journey of discovery. You will experience how easy it can be to manage your weight with herbs. Your body will reward you by becoming stronger, cleaner, and more energized. I promise you will feel the difference! Along the way, you'll gain valuable and up-to-date knowledge about herbs, spices, and whole-food meal planning.

The first section of this book is designed to provide you with the fundamental knowledge you will require to succeed at the program. By learning about the history of herbs, the anatomy and physiology of weight management, the emotional and physical aspects of working with herbs, and more, you will have a better understanding of all the many ways that herbs and herbal-based products can help you slim down so you won't have to resort to extreme, unbalanced approaches.

Master Your Metabolism provides a complete step-by-step guide to detoxifying, healing, and rejuvenating both body and mind through the proper use of herbs. This book demystifies herbs by fitting them into daily, practical use for direct results in detoxification and weight loss. It provides recipes for herbal supplements and teas based on ingredients that are easy to obtain and directions that are easy to follow. The book also shows how nutritious but inexpensive food can be prepared to rebuild and maintain vigorous good health.

I wrote this book in order to provide the public with a safe and effective herbal weight-loss system. The key to its effectiveness lies in the unusual combination of thermogenic and detoxifying herbs, essential nutrients, and foods that suppress your appetite through their rating on the Glycemic Index. These herb and food combinations boost your fat-burning metabolism and promote optimal detoxification and cleansing, helping to maintain optimal energy levels.

The herbal preparations, recipes, and meal menus in this program are designed to both detoxify and nourish. The program is designed to help you lose weight while relaxing and regenerating nerve and muscle tissue, improving cellular absorption of oxygen and other nutrients, strengthening intestinal muscles, improving peristalsis, and increasing bowel evacuation to bring about the gradual cleansing of the intestinal tract. The temperature and viscosity of the blood are normalized, thus normalizing blood pressure. These simple and natural elements of good health are arranged and indexed for easy reference and provide a unique guide to the enjoyment of good food to anyone wanting to lose weight and rid the body of toxins.

The overall result of the program is a fuller, more vigorous life. A variety of more specific results can be expected, including major improvements in digestive system functioning, reduction of arthritic pain, elimination of some types of menstrual pain, and an increase in mental concentration. The program also results in an increase in general stamina, rejuvenation of the skin, reduction in allergic reactions, increased capacity for relaxation and restful sleep, reduction and control of food cravings and mood swings, and improved mental outlook.

Each page is packed with valuable herbal and nutritional information to help you organize a complete weight-loss and health-building regimen. Some steps of the program call for ordinary fruits and vegetables, while others require easily obtained herbs, spices, grains, beans, and other ingredients. The book offers specific suggestions and guidelines to increase the vitamin, mineral, protein, and healing value of each herbal dish.

Part One of the program integrates Western and Eastern herbal healing modalities, using herbal nervines and blood cleansers along with aromatherapy and flower remedies. Much of the program involves using herbs to both cleanse the blood and increase body metabolism. Clean blood carries nutrients to the cells and removes waste from the organs and tissues. A healthy nervous system ensures proper coordination of the elimination and rebuilding functions. Part One also addresses the emotional issues connected with obesity. On a nutritional level, I address hormonal factors in obesity and explain why a high-refined carbohydrate, low-fat diet may not be the smartest choice in an effective weight-loss program.

Part Two provides the complete program, including meal plans and recipes. The herbal dietary recipes are simple to prepare, some requiring only a few minutes. Each meal will revitalize your body.

Following this program will have an immediate impact on your health and will lead you to the threshold of a greatly improved quality of life.

Chapter 1

The History of Herbal Healing

Herbal and plant remedies have been the most consistent and universal forms of treatment for human ailments for thousands of years. Plants have been the basic source of therapeutic products from prehistoric man to the early days of the twentieth century when chemotherapy (chemical-based treatments) gained popularity. More than five thousand years ago, the Sumerians had established uses for herbs. The first known book about herbs dates back to about 2700 B.C. from China and lists numerous herbs that are still used in today's modern medicine, such as ma huang, from which the common asthma drug ephedrine is derived.

Herbs and spices possess a long and illustrious history. The earliest written records indicate that teas, herbal extracts, and powders were commonly used in ancient China, India, Egypt, and Mesopotamia. Ancient Egyptian and Chinese texts record the use of herbs for treating and curing ailments of the body, mind, and spirit. The Egyptians cultivated vast herb gardens around their most important temples and their priests derived medicines from these herbs. Scholars believe that Egyptian herbalist schools existed by 3000 B.C. Even the great Pharaoh Rameses II, who died in 1225 B.C., donated more than five hundred plots of ground to be used for the cultivation of herbs after his passing.

During the biblical period, herbs were honored for their mystical and magical qualities. Essential for both medicinal and religious purposes, they were used by priests of the ancient Near East because of their secret healing powers. Many kings of biblical times used herbs for their beauty, fragrance, flavor, and therapeutic qualities. For example, King Merodaachbaladar II of Babylon, who lived during the eighth century B.C., grew more than seventy different herbs in his palace garden, and King Solomon cultivated herbs in his orchards and vineyards. According to the Roman historian Flavius Josephus, Solomon grew camphor, cinnamon, frankincense, sweet flag, aloes, lilies, and saffron.

The tradition of cataloging and describing the uses of herbs began to develop in ancient Greece, and we know of an Egyptian papyrus on the subject of herbs dating back to 1800 B.C. Many of today's culinary plants were used and described by Dioscorides, a first-century Greek physician and botanist. For fifteen hundred years, his reference work *De Materia Medica* served as the standard work on botany and the therapeutic use of plants. Before Dioscorides, there was a lack of material in ancient Greek literature on the use of herbs and spices.

As in Egypt, ancient Greek gardens were generally linked to temples. It is known, for example, that in 800 B.C. Greek priests planted herbs for therapeutic purposes in orchards surrounding the temple of Aesculapius. These priests/physicians would obtain their drugs and prepare their potions from these gardens. Known as "root-diggers," or *rhizomoi*, they gathered their herbs while offering prayers of thanksgiving.

The Greeks took the Egyptian art of aromatherapy to a more sophisticated level by planting fragrant herbs around their houses and near their living rooms. These rooms opened out onto the gardens so that when the sun shone on the plants, the fragrance of their oils would evaporate and waft into the house.

The largest expansion in herbal gardening and cultivation began with the Romans. In early Roman times, no one distinguished between ornamental and therapeutic plants. The Romans often cultivated herbs purely for their color and decoration, though some of them could also be used for medicinal and culinary purposes. The Romans created decorative herb and spice

> **Cinnamon (Cinnamomum zeylanicum):** Native to Sri Lanka, this ancient spice is still one of the most common seasonings used today. Ground cinnamon is used as a spicy sweetener in baking and cooking, as well as in beverages. Cinnamon sticks are frequently used as swizzle sticks in punches, teas, coffees, wines, and milk. Many herbalists recommend it to counter loose bowels.

gardens that were usually combinations of an orchard, vineyard, pool, and flowerbed. With the Roman conquest of Britain, herb gardening became an entrenched practice among the local peoples. Common English herbs, such as stinging nettle, were actually introduced by the Romans, who used them for many different purposes, both culinary and medicinal.

After the fall of Rome, decorative gardening faded, and gardening for foods and medicines became dominant. Most major castles had herbariums inside their walls, which proved most useful during sieges and other times when confinement were necessary.

Throughout the Middle Ages, the practice of herbology became intimately linked with astrological lore and mysticism. The planting and harvesting of herbs was influenced by the locations of the stars, and certain herbs were specifically associated with certain planets. Herbal gardening was a highly respected and widely practiced art among medieval monastic groups.

Until and throughout the twelfth century, monks within monastery walls cultivated herbs and maintained gardens with great detail. Herbs and spices were so valuable that by the ninth century, some herbs, particularly mace and cloves, were considered as valuable by some traders as gold or silver.

The monks were considered both gardeners and doctors. After harvesting and properly drying the herbs and spices, they dispensed them to the masses. Over time an inter-monastery trading system developed in which monks would trade dried herbs with distant monasteries. Monastic herb and spice gardens were usually placed near monastery infirmaries so that the fragrance of the herbs could help patients recover. It was common for monks to actually carry patients out among the fragrant herbs so that they might inhale the healing aromatic oils of these plants.

As in Greek times, there were many rites, rituals, and myths associated with the proper planting and cultivation of herbs. If a person were to ignore the specific procedures, he might be warned that nature, or the gods, would bring an undesirable fate upon him.

In the post-Medieval period, herb gardening moved out of the exclusive sphere of the monastic communities and into the newly developing scientific realm of botany. Much of this new herbology had the financial support of noblemen and European kings. Herb and spice gardens, though still important, became only a small part of much larger garden complexes that held trees, bushes, and decorative shrubs. During this period, herbs played an important role in international commerce. Much of the trade that existed between China, India, North Africa, Italy, and Spain revolved around the exchange of silks, jewels, precious goods of various types, and rare herbs and spices.

After Henry VIII broke with the Catholic Church, monasteries ceased to exist in England and English herbal gardens became completely secular. Most of these gardens followed earlier patterns of English gardens, which included walls, banks, paths, seats, fountains, and arbors.

Herb gardening was widespread on the continent from the 1500s through the 1600s. In Hamburg, Prospero Alpinus created the first public botanical garden. As a physician and professor at the University of Padua, he created the garden as a classroom to teach the true art of botany and medicine.

Herbology in the Americas

When the Spaniards began to explore the New World, they came across expansive and beautiful gardens in the fabulous Aztec capital of Tenochtitlan (present-day Mexico City). Records indicate that the Aztec king Montezuma cultivated magnificent gardens ten miles from the main city. Hernando Cortez, the famous conqueror of Mexico, described these gardens with images of color and beauty, pools and flowers, and aromatic herbs.

According to scholars, at the time of Spanish contact in 1519, more than two thousand species of medicinal plants were grown by the Aztecs in the imperial botanical gardens. The Aztecs were masters of extracting painkilling drugs from plants. Some of these were given to people before executions for crimes or as sacrifices. It is said that Montezuma's last request before his own execution was to be granted a moment in his beloved gardens. The request was honored.

Throughout the Americas, aboriginal peoples have always used herbs for healing and in spiritual rights of passage. Along with flowers, leaves, roots, and barks, medicine men used hallucinogenic mushrooms. Each tribe had its own special herbs and herbal traditions. For example, the Shoshana Indians made tea from the juniper plant, and other Native American communities used herbs for medicine, dyes, and food. These included wild blueberries, sassafras, asters, goldenrod, and wild strawberries. Many of the common fruits, vegetables, nuts, seeds, and grains we use today were common herbs among these native tribes.

The use of herbs and spices in the Americas was not limited only to native peoples. In early American history, the Puritans planted herb gardens outside of their kitchen windows. Potted herbs were grown in one half of their gardens and medicinal herbs in the other. The early American pioneers also used herbs extensively, especially lovage, sage, chives, lily of the valley, peppermint, thyme, flax, pennyroyal, and chamomile.

The Herbalist Shamans

In many cultures, the herbalist is a combination of religious leader, spiritual teacher, and medicine man. Such a person is

> **Peppermint (Mentha piperita):** is one of the most popular herbs in the world and one of the most important oils. (See the chapter on aromatherapy.) It is popular for headaches, nausea, coughs, fatigue, muscular pains, sinus congestion, apathy, digestive problems, mental tiredness, and poor circulation. Peppermint is highly effective in reducing digestive upset and has a calming effect on the emotions without the sedating quality associated with other herbs.
>
> It refreshes, restores, cools, and uplifts both body and mind. It is often added to massage blends for healing the digestive system.

known as a shaman. Many classic western images of the shaman are highly distorted. Shamans are often presented as a mixture of medicine man, gypsy tea-leaf reader, crystal ball–gazer, Oriental wise man, or mystic visionary. The hocus-pocus image of a seer who channels voices of the gods is a romantic notion that misses the point. Fundamentally, it is not what the shaman does that is so important, but rather the depth of his understanding of plants and people. Through a shaman's eyes, the individual is seen as having a spiritual destiny. On a physical level, the shaman sees the person as a complex organism containing the ability for self-healing, rather than a collection of symptoms. The shaman recognizes that illness is often an imbalance of spiritual, emotional, biochemical, and structural factors. He is able to accelerate healing by tapping into the special powers inherent in plants in order to heal what is out of balance.

Shamans believe that there is one radiant energy that pervades and gives rise to all of life that helps us to heal when we are ill. Healing herbs are especially rich in this energy. In India, this same energy is called Prana, and in Chinese medicine it is called Qi. It is believed that shamans can even communicate with some plants through an inner sixth sense. It has been said that they use their intuition to choose the right plants for use as food and medicine.

When a shaman speaks with the radiant healing energy in

plants, the line between myth and reality blurs. This radiant energy mirrors aspects of our own selves, guiding us toward our true identities, the divine reality within. The shaman does not lead a person to a spiritual dimension, but is able to give him or her the key information, herbal teas, and other plant substances to support the process.

The development of shamanic skills through the use of herbs in cooking is a celebration of the divine spark in each of us. This experience will bring joy and a sense that you are participating in the great celebration we call life while strengthening and balancing your own health. The end result is a deepened commitment to revealing the total beauty of ourselves and all of life around us. Experiencing the subtle flavors and aromas of herbs and spices is part of this process.

Herbs in Modern Medicine

Herbs and spices can be used either fresh or dried. When herbs are harvested, different parts of the plant will be gathered at different times.

Herbal products may be prepared from and include leaves, roots, oils, seeds, barks, flowers, or fruits of various trees or plants. Herbs are usually picked when they contain the highest amount of flavor essence. For example, leaves are usually picked just before the plant is about to flower; flowers are picked just before they reach full bloom; fruits and berries are picked at their peak of ripeness; and roots, like garlic, rhizomes, turmeric, and ginger, are collected in the fall, just as the leaves begin to change color.

Herbs are then packaged for health-building or culinary use. Medicinal herbs are usually available in capsule, pill, powder, or liquid form. The liquids usually consist of an extract based on alcohol, water, glycerine, apple cider vinegar, or a combination of these extracting agents.

Today, spices in food, as well as herbal teas, baths, salves, and ointments, are more popular than ever for bringing relief from illness. They have recently become even more popular as a tool in weight-management programs. Today, as much as 75 percent of all pharmaceutical drugs contain plant-derived substances or variations of plant compounds. Examples include red rice yeast for reducing high cholesterol; aspirin, a synthetic variation on salicylic acid, which was discovered in white willow bark; St. John's Wort, which is recommended for depression; black cohosh, red clover, and soy for menopause; hawthorn berries for congestive heart disease; saw palmetto for prostatitis; and ginkgo leave extracts for Alzheimer's disease.

Numerous studies have shown that certain herbs can reduce appetite and increase the body's metabolic rate. These are two factors that are key elements to most successful weight-management programs.

Although there is now more sophisticated research on the value of herbal medicines than ever before, most of the information on herbs used in weight management and food preparation is based on folklore passed down from generation to generation. Over the past fifteen years, the use of many culinary herbs and spices as healing medicines has increased to an amazing level because of:

1. A desire amongst people to live a more natural lifestyle
2. A fear of the side effects associated with many over-the-counter and prescription drugs, heightened by recent scares related to weight-loss drugs used at professional dieting centers
3. Dissatisfaction with the high cost and impersonal style of orthodox medicine
4. The effect of the movement toward multiculturalism, which has caused a refocusing on the importance of herbal medicine in Indian, African, Asian, and South American cultures

Though herbs may not act as quickly on the body as drugs do, many people experience a qualitative as well as a quantitative difference in favor of herbs.

Hawthorn (Crataegus spp.): Native to England and Europe, it is most prized for its fruit (berry) and for extracts from its leaves. Hawthorn is one of the most researched cardiotonic plants in the world. Known for reducing blood pressure, it also improves blood flow to and through the heart and improves metabolic processes in the myocardium. The first recorded use of hawthorn was in the first century A.D. by the Greek herbalist Dioscorides. The value for hawthorn in weight management is that it contains significant thermogenic properties.

The berries, leaves, and flowers of hawthorn contain a variety of bioflavonoid-like complexes (including oligomeric procyanidins, vitexin, and hyperoside), which appear to be primarily responsible for its cardiac benefits. These same bioflavonoids are also sources of potent antioxidants. Extracts of both leaves and flowers are widely used in Europe.

Herbs and spices are among the most versatile foods and healing tools in nature. They can be used in oil form or in powders, pills, and liquids. They can be prepared fresh, sprouted, cooked, and can even be juiced. Not only do they have a naturally detoxifying and cleansing effect on the body and mind, but they also help purify the blood and the internal organs, neutralize the waste products of metabolism, and help in building new healthy tissue

The beneficial effect of herbs and spices in the resolution of many health problems is attributed to the following physiological facts:

1. Herbs and spices are rich in many essential nutrients, especially vitamins, minerals, trace elements, and enzymes.
2. Fresh herbs and spices provide an alkaline surplus that is extremely important for normalizing the acid-alkaline ratio in the blood and tissues. Excessive acidity is present in many conditions of ill health and is considered to be a contributing factor in the development of many diseases.

3. Herbs and spices speed the recovery from disease by supplying needed substances for the body's own healing activity and cell regeneration.

4. Many of the vital nutritive elements in herbs are assimilated directly through the tissues of the mouth into the blood stream, without putting a strain on the digestive system.

5. Mineral imbalance in the tissues is one of the main causes of diminished oxygenation, which may lead to premature aging of cells and disease. The generous amounts of easily assimilated organic minerals, particularly the calcium, potassium, and silicon that is in some herbs, can help to restore biochemical and mineral balance in the tissues and cells.

6. Herbs, spices, and different vegetal hormones and antibiotics are contained in nature's own medicines. String beans, for example, are known to contain insulin-like substances; cucumbers and onions contain hormones essential for the pancreas; and antibiotic substances are present in fresh garlic, onions, radish, and tomatoes.

7. Research has shown that raw herbs, fruits, and vegetables contain an as-yet unidentified factor that is responsible for the cell's ability to absorb nutrients from the blood stream and effectively excrete metabolic wastes from the cell.

8. The various coloring substances—red, yellow, green, and blue—in all shades and intensities, which are present in fruits, vegetables, and herbs, increase production of red blood corpuscles, influence digestive and assimilative processes, and take part in the metabolism of proteins and cholesterol.

9. Lycopene, a natural antioxidant found exclusively in tomatoes, is getting much attention in the press as a cancer fighter. In the early 1990s, tomatoes and tomato-based products were spotlighted as potentially preventative. In studies conducted at Harvard, forty-eight thousand health professionals were followed for six years and monitored for

evidence of prostate cancer. Researchers read the results to suggest that lycopene might decrease the risk of prostate cancer, whereas other dietary antioxidants, including beta-carotene, appeared to have no effect. (Levine).

It is easy to see, from the above, why plant foods, especially herbs, spices, fruits, and vegetables, have such an important role to play in this weight-management program.

Why Herbal and Whole-Food Concentrate Supplementation Is Recommended

Whole-food concentrates are nutrient-rich products generally in the form of liquids, powders, tablets, or capsules. They are combinations of dehydrated juices, whole foods, and herbal products. They are favored by those consumers who see the value of nutritional supplementation, but who want to limit their intake of synthetic ingredients even in their nutritional supplementation. The essential nutrients in these products are lower in dosage than traditional vitamin/mineral supplements, but whole-food concentrates are more easily absorbed by many people and are beneficial under the following circumstances:

1. If you have poor dietary habits, malabsorption, or past nutritional deficiencies
2. If you are on a calorie-restricted diet
3. If you use birth control pills
4. If you are avoiding certain foods to reduce your fat intake
5. If you smoke
6. If you are under considerable physical or emotional stress
   Stress can use up large amounts of dietary nutrients, as well as the body's stored-up vital enzymes and other biochemicals.
7. If you drink alcohol on a regular basis
   Alcohol destroys vitamin B2 and B6, folic acid, and vitamins A, C, and D; it also flushes minerals out of the system.
8. If you are facing a major medical stress, such as serious burns, major surgery, or cancer

By combining an herbal-based weight-management program with healthy herbal cooking, you become part of a long and illustrious tradition. The use of herbs and spices lies at the heart of the history of medicine and healing, as well as at the center of whole-foods cookery. Here is an opportunity to experience a cornucopia of scents, colors, and textures while shedding excess weight in the process.

Chapter 2

The Anatomy and Physiology of Weight Loss

Obesity is one of the greatest health problems affecting our society, and the selling of weight-loss products including books, tapes, and special supplements is one of the fastest-growing industries in America.

Obviously, the solution for those of us who are overweight or even obese is to lose weight. However, weight loss doesn't take place just by cutting calories or dietary fat reduction. It's more complex than that. Whether someone is slim or heavy is influenced by many factors including genetics, endocrinology, and neurology, as well as childhood nutritional patterns. Walk down any supermarket aisle, and you will be confronted with seemingly unlimited choices of processed, pre-packaged foods of every type imaginable, many with the words "natural" on the label. No matter how these foods are labeled, they often have two things in common: they are high in fat and low in fiber. These two factors alone are the cause of much of the obesity in America. One of the great benefits of an herbal-based nutrition program is that it is low in fat and high in fiber. My own program includes some herbs that serve as appetite suppressants and others that inhibit the accumulation of fat.

A whopping 65 percent of Americans start new diets at least once a year. Study after study shows that Americans are the fattest people on the planet, and getting fatter still. There are more than twenty-eight diets on public record, and yet, despite our apparent mental obsession with dieting, we display no corresponding obsession with proper dietary habits. As a result, obesity may be the greatest single health risk we face as a nation today.

What is obesity? When a person takes in more calories than he or she uses, the excess calories are stored as fat. Fat, or adipose cells, have the ability to expand or contract based on how a specific body uses energy. Most people usually define their degree of obesity by stepping on a scale or by measuring the thickness of a fold of skin around the triceps, shoulder blades, or hips.

But you may be overweight even though standard height-weight charts tell you that you are within the "normal" range. And as you age, the way your body holds fat will change, sometimes with drastic results. For example, a man who weighed 150 pounds for twenty years may not have been overweight twenty years ago, but he could be overweight today if his weight has settled around his midsection.

As a rule of thumb, if you are carrying 25 percent or more of your body weight in fat, then you are obese. Here is a quick method for determining whether you are in a "safe" weight range: if you are an adult male, your chest should be at least 5 inches larger than your waist. If you are an adult female, your chest should be 10 inches larger than your waist.

For some very obese people, going on a long-term, low-calorie diet may result in very limited weight loss. The reason is that their metabolic rate may drop to "protect" them from starvation. As anyone loses weight, their body requires fewer calories. To continue losing weight at the same pace, therefore, a person must lower their caloric intake. "For example, a moderately active female weighing 135 pounds can lose about a pound a week on a fifteen hundred calorie diet. Once down to 124 pounds, however, she must consume no more than twelve hundred calories a day to maintain this rate of loss," (Dartnell Corporation).

The sanest approach to losing weight is to use a nutritionally balanced, healthy, herbal-based weight-loss program. I say healthy because there are many controversial herbal formulas on the market that derive their effectiveness from overstimulating the central nervous system. Some of the most commonly used herbal weight-loss products are effective because of the stimulating effects they have on mental and physical functions. Many of these herbal products contain stimulants such as caffeine or ephedrine. Most are promoted as "natural" alternatives to the controversial prescription drug combination commonly known as "fen-phen."

The anti-obesity prescription drugs dexfenfluramine (brand name Redux) and fenfluramine (brand name Pondimin), were withdrawn from the marketplace because of consumer complaints concerning their safety.

The key ingredients of most herbal fen-phen products are ephedra (found in the herb ma huang) and caffeine. Ephedra is a powerful stimulant and thermogenic compound (a compound that helps the body burn brown adipose tissue) with the potential to affect the nervous system and heart. When used properly, they are generally safe, but unfortunately many people, desperate to lose weight, overuse them, which can lead to health problems including high blood pressure, heart rate irregularities, insomnia, nervousness, tremors, headaches, seizures, heart attacks, and strokes.

Caffeinated herbs have been used throughout history and seem to pop up in just about every culture. Of course, coffee, tea, and cocoa are the most familiar of these in modern times. Among the most popular of these stimulants are kola nut, bissy nut, guarana, yerba maté, and tea. Many herbalists do not approve of the regular use of stimulants as a tool for weight loss.

A number of the medical problems most associated with general obesity and stress-induced obesity might be aggravated by even moderate intake of caffeinated products. Persons with active heart disease, hypertension (high blood pressure), and gastric ulcers should be particularly aware.

According to the *Physicians' Desk Reference for Nonprescription Drugs*, over-consumption of caffeine, even by the ordinary consumer, can cause nervousness, sleeplessness, irritability, anxiety, and/or heart palpitations.

The most effective and the safest weight-loss products combine "anti-fat" nutrients with herbs that will maximize weight loss. Effective and safe programs also curb or eliminate lipogenesis (the process by which your body produces and stores fat), cut sugar and carbohydrate cravings, control your appetite, suppress food intake, burn stored fat without loss of lean body mass, and increase your energy level.

The Four Most Common Myths about Losing Weight with Herbs

1. There is a magic herbal pill that will simply make you lose weight, make pounds melt away, or burn fat. No such herb exists.
2. You can lose weight in a few weeks, and if you keep taking herbal weight-loss products it will stay off.
3. You can lose weight permanently by fasting.
4. All fat is bad. In fact, some fat is essential in your diet. Fat serves as a shock absorber for your internal organs, and it is a good source of stored energy. Most of all it is required to absorb vitamins A, D, E, and K, the fat-soluble vitamins.

Ten Dieting Traps and Why They Must Be Avoided

As you move toward healthy weight loss using my herbal method, remember that just about any diet has the potential to help you lose weight, but the real challenge is to keep it off. How does one do this? Stay away from fad diets and compulsive patterns. If you want to lose weight for good, avoid skipping meals. Skipping meals may lead to bingeing later on.

When evaluating your weight, it is best to avoid scales or the type of weight charts issued by insurance companies. Most important is not how fat you are, but what your fat/lean body-mass ratio is. It is body composition that counts, not just fat.

Body composition can be determined by a number of ways, including skin fold calipers, infrared measurements, and bioimpedance machines. Any physician or properly trained fitness instructor can do this measurement for you, or you can learn to do it yourself. Most of all, eat a variety of healthy foods. Because fad diets often recommend large amounts of a specific food (i.e. all protein or all apples), they deprive your body of essential nutrients and lack variety and balance. Beware of diets that promote this kind of unbalanced weight loss. Almost any food can be used to excess. Those people who tend toward excessive or compulsive eating patterns often seek out one miracle food to magically burn the fat off of their body. Unfortunately, they are always disappointed. Some of the healthiest, most nutritious foods can become problematic if used in excess, or if eaten as part of a nutritionally deficient program. Here are a few areas to be aware of.

1. Do not begin a weight-loss program before you're emotionally ready. It is important that you are highly motivated to begin and maintain your weight-management program. If you are not committed to this process, the weight loss won't last for long. For support in this area see chapter 7—Flower Remedies.

2. Beware of rigid menus and nutritionally unbalanced weight-loss diets. Few people follow diets that require strict adherence to rigid menus for any reasonable length of time. Even if they start off with the best intentions, boredom and frustration usually win out in the end. This can lead to eating an unbalanced diet in a misguided quest to cut back on calories and/or fat. Some people cut out entire food groups, such as grains or carbohydrates.

3. Beware of magic herbal formulas. Diets that claim that certain foods or herbal pills will magically make fat disappear without any special calorie-control programs are not worth following. Avoid at all costs.

4. Beware of the "promise you everything" diets. Diets that promise that you will lose large amounts of weight overnight should arouse your natural suspicion. Keep this in mind: at the beginning of virtually any diet that restricts calories and carbohydrates, the weight you lose is water. That's right. Water! And studies show that the faster you lose weight, the more likely you are to regain it. Most gimmicky fad diets work in the short run because they are low in calories, not because of anything special about the diet.

5. Don't expect to magically lose weight. Don't trust a program that sounds too good to be true. You are not going to lose fourteen pounds in ten days and do so in a way that does not put stress on your body. Fat does not melt away while you sleep. You lose weight by exercising, reducing caloric intake, and increasing your metabolism in a balanced and healthy way.

6. Beware of keeping your shelves empty. Keep healthy snacking foods around the house. Because they're afraid of overeating, many people who are trying to lose weight keep little or no food in their cupboards.

7. Beware of blaming your set point. The "set point" theory suggests that your body "wants" to be a particular weight. Some overweight people use this as an excuse for not trying to drop excess pounds. But you can set realistic goals, such as losing 10 percent of your weight (twenty pounds if you weigh two hundred pounds). Maintain this weight for six months, and if you still want to lose more, give it a try.

8. Beware of extreme protein diets. According to a report in the *Tufts University Diet & Nutrition Newsletter* (March 1985), in spite of the recent proliferation of high-fat, high-protein diets, most nutritional experts agree that there is too much, rather than too little, protein in the typical American diet. In other words, excessively high protein

intake can cause the body to lose calcium through the urine. In the long run, especially in the elderly, this calcium loss can place some individuals at greater risk for the brittle bones and unexpected fractures associated with osteoporosis. Beware of diets that use excessively high or low amounts of protein. Ingesting overly high levels of protein will increase your risk of many serious illnesses, including cancer and heart disease. Other side effects can include constipation, cramps, bad breath, and hair loss. When your diet is too low in protein, your body may damage itself by utilizing the protein from your own organs and muscles.

9. Beware of diets that recommend less than one thousand calories per day. When you cut your caloric intake suddenly, your body may reduce the number of calories it burns. Thus you may follow a low-calorie diet and still not lose weight.

10. Beware of fasting. Fasting alone, and fasting combined with an herbal detoxification program, can be a very powerful healing tool, but it may not be the most effective approach to weight control. This is because people who lose weight through fasting not only lose body fat, but also lean muscle tissue. The loss of lean muscle mass can result in a reduction in a person's basal-metabolic rate that makes it more difficult for them to continue to lose weight and maintain the weight loss they have already achieved. In addition to this problem, when a fasting dieter puts the weight back on, it is primarily as fat. If a person begins to yo-yo diet, the long-term effect will be an increased difficulty in losing weight and regaining pounds already lost. Another problem with fasting as a weight-loss strategy is that extremely low-fat diets can actually increase blood levels of certain types of "undesirable cholesterol." If fasting isn't the most effective path, then what is?

The four most important herbal and dietary factors in an effective weight-loss program are:

- Designing an effective and balanced herbal system
- Choosing foods properly
- Eating moderately
- Increasing the body's metabolism, especially through the effective use of thermogenic herbs. Fasting alone does not help you practice any of these four. A well-balanced herbal detoxification program can, however, increase nutrient absorption while increasing metabolism. Thus a semi-herbal fast does have value in this way.

11. Beware of going from one diet to another within a short period of time. Avoid making too many changes at once. Some people will start on a high-fat, low-carbohydrate diet. Then they switch to a diet that cuts back drastically on fat and calories and increases fruits and vegetables. Then they switch to an intense daily exercise and juice program. All this switching can set you up for failure.

12. Beware of thinking that weight-loss drugs are a solution. Weight-loss medications like sibutramine (Meridia) and listat (Xenical) are generally reserved for those whose excess weight poses a threat to health. Work with a nutritionally trained holistic physician if necessary before you consider the drug route to weight loss.

The Primary Causes of Obesity

There is no one cause of obesity. Some people are more easily able to identify the reasons why they are unable to lose weight and keep it off once they have lost it. For some individuals, the origin of the weight gain was a basic shift in lifestyle. They may have gotten married, had a work-related injury, experienced cultural pressure, had poor exercise patterns or changed their exercise patterns due to a sports injury, had a baby, or quit smoking. For others it is hereditary factors. It may be a medical problem with neurological regulators or natural hormonal factors such as thyroid gland dysfunction. It may also be a digestive disorder, blood sugar disease (hypoglycemia or diabetes), enzymatic activity, brain mechanisms, genetic predisposition, or they may simply take in more calories from the food that they eat than they expend. Let's take a closer look at a few of these factors and how an effective herbal weight program might reduce their influence.

Enzymatic Activity

The enzyme lipoprotein lipase (LPL) is a factor that may influence obesity. LPL helps the body store excess calories in fat cells. The enzyme is manufactured in fat cells and is transported to the capillaries, where it breaks dietary fat into tiny particles that penetrate the membranes of these fat cells. The process becomes a vicious cycle of cells continuously collecting fat and LPL levels rising, which causes more fat to be collected from the bloodstream. Reducing caloric intake decreases LPL levels, but when a person begins to overeat or even return to normal meal patterns, LPL levels may become higher than before the diet began. Using herbs, such as Garcinia cambogia extract and Gymnema sylvestre, can naturally reduce the tendency to overeat and thus reduce the factors that cause an increase in LPL levels.

Brain Mechanisms

Many obesity experts believe that there is a mechanism in the brain known as the adipostat, which tells the body how much fat to store. This is, in turn, based on a predefined weight that the body wishes to maintain. As your body uses fat through your daily activities, the brain regulates the usage or storage of energy until your fat levels maintain this preestablished goal. Sometimes the adipostat may actually set a fat storage level that is unhealthy. In such a case, simply reducing your caloric intake may not reduce weight so easily. While you may be cutting back on fat and calories, the brain may be sabotaging your efforts by restoring your original, excess weight by causing you to consume more calories due to hunger sensations.

There is a belief among many researchers that there is a specific hormone in the body known as HGH (human growth hormone), which helps people to burn fat and build muscle. HGH is present at high levels in children so that they convert fat quickly into muscle and meet the needs of rapidly growing bodies. Research has indicated that this fat-burning hormone is released at a slower pace as a person reaches thirty years old and virtually stops after thirty. Nutritional scientists also believe that this hormone is dormant in individuals who are plagued by obesity whatever their age. The body stores HGH in the pituitary gland and releases it in response to sleep, exercise, fasting, and by the amino acids L-arginine, L-ornithine, and L-lysine.

Through metabolic and behavioral regulation, the pituitary and adrenal glands control eating patterns. They are able to recognize and respond to certain signals that indicate hunger or the existence of high-fat storage in the body. How the body recognizes this key information is defined by numerous variables. One of these variables is leptin. Leptin is an enzyme that signals the brain when fat storage is high. Fat cells release leptin; levels rise as more fat is stored in the cells. If fat storage falls, then lower leptin levels signal to stimulate appetite. Certain herbs have been shown to influence the regulation of metabolic and behavioral patterns.

Genetic Factors

Though it is unlikely a "fat" gene causes obesity, there is evidence that a number of genetic factors may influence people most likely to be obese. LPL activity, metabolic rates, hormonal fluctuations in response to the changing of the seasons, distribution of fat, food preferences, and other factors may be influenced by genetics and in turn increase the chances of obesity.

And then there are emotional factors. Many people deal with their anxiety, or rather don't deal with it, by eating. They raid the cookie jar or the refrigerator when they feel sad, abandoned, or depressed. Eating is often used as a way to stifle feelings rather than acknowledge them. The use of flower remedies and aro-

Licorice (Glycyrrhiza glabra): Licorice is a perennial plant native to southern Europe and Asia. This ancient Egyptian cure-all is also called *liquorice*, meaning "the sweet root." Its roots and rhizomes are prized both medicinally and for their sweet flavoring. Bladder, stomach, and kidney problems also respond favorably to licorice, and it can relieve thirst as well as satisfy a desire for candy, sweets, and cigarettes. Licorice tones and maintains health of the adrenal cortex. In folklore remedies, it is recommended for the treatment of hypoglycemia, though probably only when this is caused by adrenocortical insufficiency, and especially when stress is the main cause of the adrenal insufficiency.

In the Caribbean, many parents give their children licorice sticks to chew on in place of candy. Licorice has been unfairly maligned of late, probably because of a perceived connection with candy store licorice, with which it has no relation at all. Licorice root is available in many natural food stores and in ethnic spice shops. Among its various uses, licorice sticks make great swizzle sticks for drinks.

matherapy have become powerful tools for balancing out those emotions that might lead to overeating. Curbing obesity has its definite advantages. According to recent studies, "For many obese people, relatively small weight losses—say, only 10 percent of body weight—can correct a tendency toward diabetes or high blood pressure." ("Research Lifts Blame") Thus losing only ten to twenty-five pounds can help avert major health risks.

Poor nutrition is the greatest culprit in a majority of weight problems. Knowing the basic facts about obesity, nutrition, and dieting will provide you with the necessary background information you need to begin a truly successful and healthy diet.

Isolating the Cause

Once the cause is isolated and corrected, losing weight and keeping it off becomes a simple process of exercise, food management,

Flax: Many people suffering from obesity starve themselves and/or restrict their diet to non-fat or low-fat foods only to find that they gain weight or remain the same. If only they knew that one of the best ways to fight fat is with fat!

Believe it or not, one of the most effective ways to lose weight naturally is by consuming unsaturated fats, such as flaxseed oil. The unhealthy fats are saturated fats, which contribute to cardio-vascular disease, strokes, obesity, and other degenerative diseases. But flaxseed oil can be considered an anti-fat or non-fat fat because it prevents, and in some cases reverses, the effects of saturated fat in the body.

Flaxseed oil works with the physiologic and metabolic processes in the body. The human body requires fatty acids in order to function properly, and the fatty acids found in flaxseed oil have been found to be essential nutrients. The body cannot convert other food sources into these essential fatty acids. To get them, you have to consume flaxseed oil.

Adding flaxseed oil your meals will make you feel fuller longer and will decrease your craving for sweets and fatty foods because your body will be getting the essential nutrients it needs.

Flaxseed oil also helps to regulate blood sugar and insulin levels. The essential fats in flaxseed oil keep food in the stomach longer. This causes a gradual increase, a sustained plateau, and finally a gradual decrease of blood sugar. Because your body doesn't have to combat a sharp rise in blood sugar, often found after the consumption of low or non-fat foods, insulin levels will be more regulated. The overall effect will be one of increased energy, stamina, and mental clarity, and a feeling of longer-lasting satiation.

The body breaks down flaxseed oil into compounds that boost the metabolic rate in cells. Because the cells work faster, more heat is created, resulting in the burning of more calories. Flaxseed oil increases aerobic function (oxygen consumption) in the cells, which also facilitates weight loss, increases energy and stamina, and promotes a general feeling of well-being.

Flaxseed oil not only is useful for weight loss, but also helps detoxify the body by improving liver function.

To benefit most from the uses of flaxseed oil, I suggest that you take one to two tablespoons daily. For the maximum benefit in weight loss and maintenance, it is recommended that this amount be divided and a portion taken with each meal.

and naturally increasing the body's metabolic rate. This is an approach that can be useful and effective, even for the chronically obese. For these individuals, weight loss is a difficult process no matter what they eat, and no matter how hard they try. The cause may be a chemical imbalance in the appetite control centers of the brain, genetics, or some unknown factor. An herbal weight-management program is especially of value for these individuals, since they are at a higher risk for medical conditions associated with obesity. They are at increased risk for developing maturity onset diabetes, high blood pressure, degenerative joint disease (osteoarthritis, etc.), cardiovascular disease (heart attacks, strokes, etc.), and numerous other medical problems. Here are nine primary causes of obesity.

1. A calorie-restricted diet from which you may not be getting adequate nutrients
2. Bad eating habits, nutritional deficiencies, or malabsorption
2. Excessive emotional or physical stress
3. Smoking
4. Drinking alcohol regularly
6. Food intolerance or sensitivity reactions
7. Heading into, being in the middle of, or recovering from any major medical stress such as surgery or cancer treatment
8. Taking birth control pills
9. Having any psychological disorder, particularly depression

One Calorie Does Not Always Equal One Calorie

Are all calories equal? Does it matter whether you intake one calorie from a fat or one calorie from a carbohydrate?

For years, some experts argued that all calories are equal. But experts now admit it is much more complex than that. "Only about 1 percent of ingested carbohydrates end up as body fat," as opposed to 2.5 percent for ingested fats. Therefore, one calorie from fat is less efficient for weight loss than one calorie from a starch. As a result, simply switching from a high-fat diet to one high in carbohydrates, without actually lowering total caloric intake, can result in a net caloric loss to the body ("Research Lifts Blame").

Remember: as you lose weight, your body requires fewer calories. So to continue losing weight at the pace you want, you may need to lower your caloric intake altogether.

Health Problems and Obesity

Obesity paves the way for a wide range of health problems. It weakens the abdominal muscles, placing greater stress on the back muscles, and makes it harder to maintain the body in an upright position. Other ailments that obesity can contribute to, or aggravate, include gallbladder disease, hypertension, arthritis, and reduced immune-system response.

Obesity and the Nutritional Fundamentals

There are many nutrients essential for good health. Our bodies can manufacture some nutrients, and others can only be obtained from our food. The nutrients that must come from food are called the essential nutrients. These are protein, fats, carbohydrates, vitamins, minerals, and water. How much of each of these is needed in relation to the others is the source of most controversy in the field of nutrition, and in the promoting of various weight-loss programs.

Protein

We all know that adequate protein is necessary to ensure physical well-being, but in the last several decades its importance has been exaggerated. A protein intake as high as 150 grams a day has been proposed, but it can be said that anything over seventy grams a day is too high. A daily protein intake of thirty to fifty grams is what most people actually require, although those who engage in heavy physical labor or sports may require more. If a high protein intake brings excessive caloric intake with it then an unnecessary weight gain may result.

Proteins:
1. Restore and renew body tissue and cells
2. Ensure proper distribution of fluids throughout the body
3. Maintain body functions and create antibodies for the immune system

Fats

Fats are complex combinations of what we call lipids, fatty substances that include fat-soluble vitamins, tocopherols, triglycerides, sterols, and phospholipids. Each fat or oil has its own combination of these substances, which is why each fat or oil has its own distinct flavor, melting point, burning point, and texture.

Many people think of fat as something undesirable, unhealthy, and bad. But there are many types of fat. There are good and bad dietary fats. Good dietary fat is not only good, but is essential for health. For instance, fats provide essential fatty acids that assist body cells in the reception and absorption of fat-soluble vitamins A, D, E, and K.

All kinds of problems result from inadequate good fat and too much bad fat, from dandruff to depression. In addition to dietary fats, there are liquid and aromatic fats that are not dietary, but are extremely valuable nonetheless for healing and weight loss. These are the aromatic oils that are essential to the practice of aromatherapy. These are discussed later on throughout this program.

As for nutrition, the body requires certain fats, or components of fats, for proper functioning. These fats supply essential fatty acids needed for innumerable glandular and metabolic processes. They also provide twice as much energy as carbohydrates. Many of these essential fatty acids are abundant in certain fish oils and in the seeds of certain herbs. Though I think essential fatty acid supplementation is valuable, I recommend borage and evening primrose oil over fish oil supplements for three reasons.

1. It is possible that fish oils might be contaminated with PCBs (polychlorinated bi-phenyls) or other pollutants. Though reputable companies should have quality control to prevent this problem I would rather use plant sources for these oils.

2. Excessive intake of fish oils could result in an increased need for vitamin E and bleeding problems.

3. People have been known to experience vitamin A or D toxicity from excessive use of fish-liver oil.

Research shows that the essential omega 3 fatty acids can be obtained from vegetable and plant sources without any of the potential risk factors associated with fish oil.

Saturated fat is solid fat at room temperature. Unsaturated fat is fat that is liquid at room temperature and is called oil. Animal fat is usually saturated and vegetable fat is usually unsaturated. Some vegetable fats are saturated, as they are solid or semi-solid at room temperature. Examples are coconut oils and palm kernal oils. The less a fat has been processed and the fresher it is, the more likely its important elements will survive to fill the body's needs.

All fats are to some extent processed. Fats that have been highly processed—by extraction and preparation methods that heat them or otherwise cause changes in their molecular structure—should be avoided.

Some individuals, in an attempt to reduce their intake of animal fat, will remove butter from their diet and replace it with cholesterol-free oil. Since margarine is made from vegetable rather then animal sources, they have come to believe that polyunsaturated oils are lower in fat or are somehow healthier for them. Nothing could be further from the truth. These are highly undesirable, synthetic products that have been hydrogenated (the

Borage Seed Oil (Borago officinalis): Borage oil is extracted by what is called expeller pressing from the seeds of the borage herb. This oil, as is evening primrose oil, is rich in gamma-linolenic acid and linoleic acid, both essential omega 6 fatty acids. Borage oil is the richest natural source of gamma-linolenic acid. Gamma-linolenic acid is very useful as a direct precursor of type 1-prostaglandins. These prostaglandins are essential for good activity of the skin cells. These functions concern not only skin tissues, but also the nervous tissue, the circulatory system, and the reproductive organs.

A supplement of borage oil is useful in cases of skin troubles (premature wrinkles, lack of elasticity), to fight against aging of tissues, and nervous troubles (stress, anxiety). Borage oil can be applied externally by piercing the capsule with a needle, then spreading on the face and the other parts of the skin that need to be treated (wrinkles, eczema, dry areas, stretch marks, etc.).

adding of hydrogen to created the hardening effect), and usually contain large amounts of artificial flavors, colors, and preservatives as well as produce unhealthy by-products known as trans-fatty acids.

There is one type of fat that is neither saturated nor unsaturated, but is wholly unnatural and is impossible for the body to metabolize. This is called hydrogenated fat. Good unsaturated fat, such as corn oil, is solidified by hydrogenization, the addition of hydrogen to harden the liquid oil. The resulting product cannot be digested effectively, creating a trans-fatty acid that can cause heart disease. Hydrogenated fats are added to many commercially prepared foods. Margarine is one of the more common examples. Avoid any food that says, "partially hydrogenated," "hydrogenated," or "partially hardened" on the label.

In addition to saturated, unsaturated, and polyunsaturated fats, there are monounsaturated fats. These include olive oil and some fish oils, which are quite beneficial. They decrease LDL

> **Grapeseed Oil:** Grapeseed oil is a high-linoleic acid product. Linoleic acid is one of two essential fatty acids your body cannot manufacture—you must take it in through dietary sources. It is the only food known to raise HDL and lower LDL. You may know linoleic acid as omega 6. Studies indicate that linoleic acid is sadly deficient in our diets. Grapeseed oil is 76 percent linoleic acid! It is valuable for those looking to lose weight because it not only helps to prevent hypertension caused by sodium excess, but also helps to normalize lesions occurring from obesity and diabetes leading to heart disease. Grapeseed oil can be used for salad dressing and in cooking. It has a non-greasy, slightly nutty flavor. An article in *American College of Cardiology,* (March 14–18, 1993) indicates that grapeseed oil is best for heart-health ranking, above olive oil and canola oil.

cholesterol in the blood while protecting the blood level of HDL cholesterol. LDL is low-density lipoprotein. This kind of cholesterol is associated with the accumulation of arterial plaque, which causes narrowing of the arteries and can lead to the increased likelihood of a heart attack. HDL is high-density lipoprotein. This kind of cholesterol is beneficial, because your body can use it for primary functions. Current research is showing that when it comes to fat, the real issue at hand is not simply saturated or unsaturated fat, but rather the level of essential omega 3 and omega 6 fatty acids in a person's diet.

Though deficiencies of essential fatty acids were thought to be rare, experts are beginning to suggest that the condition may be more widespread than previously thought. Many people who exhibit the symptoms listed below have been found to have abnormally low blood and/or tissue levels of these essential fatty acids.

Linoleic acid—Behavioral changes, thirst, abnormal water loss through the skin, kidney degeneration, hair loss, arthritis, heart problems, circulatory problems, poor wound healing, poor growth, miscarriage in females, sterility in males, reduced immunity, eczema type skin eruptions, gallbladder problems, prostatitis, acne, and muscle tremors.

Linolenic acid—Poor growth, impaired vision, impaired learning ability, poor motor coordination, and tingling in the legs and arms.

All of these symptoms will clear up if appropriate amounts of essential fatty acids (EFAs) are returned to the diet. Good sources of EFAs are canola oil, flaxseed oil, borage oil, walnut oil, and good old monounsaturated olive oil.

How to Choose Healthy Fats and Oils

1. Avoid foods that have been fried. Broil, bake, or steam your food whenever possible. Steaming is superior to boiling because there is less nutrient loss.
2. Limit your use of eggs and poultry.
3. Limit your intake of fats and oils, especially foods high in saturated fat. These include butter, cream, lard, heavily hydrogenated fats, many margarines, shortenings, and foods containing palm and/or coconut oils.
4. Limit the amount of oil you use in food preparation, and when you do use oil, always choose flaxseed oil, pumpkin-seed oil, walnut oil, canola oil, or extra-virgin olive oil that has been cold pressed.
5. Choose dry beans, peas (in combination with whole grains), or low-fat, fermented milk products (yogurt, kefir, etc.) as protein sources rather than beef, pork, and whole-milk products.

Complex Carbohydrates

Unrefined complex carbohydrates are the best source of energy for a healthy body and are an extremely important part of a weight-management program. They are essential for the functioning of your brain and nervous system, supply energy for digestion and muscular exertion, and are necessary for proper absorption of other foods. By providing this type of energy,

Evening Primrose Oil (Oenothera biennis lamarkiana): This oil is extracted from the seeds of the evening primrose plant. This oil is generally extracted from this plant by simple pressure without the use of heat or solvents. This herbally derived oil is a polyunsaturated oil that is the richest source of the essential omega 6 fatty acids: linoleic acid and gamma-linolenic acid.

Gamma-linolenic acid (GLA), an essential fatty acid, is the active ingredient in both borage and evening primrose oils. It is a precursor of prostaglandins, a shortage of which may cause the mood changes and cramping experienced by many women suffering from PMS. This fatty acid may improve nerve function in diabetics.

Unfortunately, many variables may inhibit the production of GLA and prostaglandins. Among the inhibiting factors are cholesterol, old age, radiation, chemical carcinogens, alcohol, and saturated fats. EPO has the ability to lower blood cholesterol, lower blood pressure to normal, and help lower excess weight without dieting. EPO has been shown to be one hundred times more effective than other polyunsaturated oils in lowering cholesterol.

Evening primrose oil can be especially useful for women trying to lose weight who are experiencing the symptoms of premenstrual syndrome. Premenstrual syndrome disrupts the life of many women, and it is hard to imagine a person focusing on their eating habits when they are experiencing headaches, migraines, painful tension in the breasts, bowel problems, irritability, and anxiety. Recent research has indicated that these symptoms can be traced to a deficiency of gamma-linolenic and linoleic acids. In the past, the ordinary vegetable oil used in food would have provided linoleic acid. But the increasingly technological manufacturing process and cooking have altered it to such an extreme level that the organism is unable to produce type-1 prostaglandin with it. By taking some natural elements necessary to produce these prostaglandins, linoleic and gamma-linolenic acids, you may avoid premenstrual syndrome troubles. Since evening primrose oil is 72 percent linoleic acid and 10 percent gamma-linolenic acid, it is an ideal nutritional supplement.

In addition to premenstrual problems, this oil has also been shown to be effective in treating hormonal troubles and circulatory troubles such as varicose veins and hemorrhoids. All of these are conditions that are sometimes related to obesity and excessive weight.

Studies have shown that evening primrose oil has the ability to:

1. Lower blood pressure to normal
2. Lower blood cholesterol
3. Lower weight in the overweight without dieting

carbohydrates actually lessen the body's requirement for protein to perform these functions. Your body is then free to use any protein you consume for the repairing of damaged tissue and for building new, healthy tissue.

In spite of all the recent controversy surrounding fats vs. carbohydrates in weight management, most nutritional experts agree that in attempting to reduce your weight to "ideal" levels, unrefined complex carbohydrates have one key advantage over fats: they contain less than half the number of calories per ounce than fats. Complex carbohydrates are also valuable for purification and detoxification through their ability to help the body convert certain chemicals, bacterial toxins, and some normal metabolites (the end-products of the physical and chemical processes involved in the maintenance of life) into a form that can be easily eliminated as waste.

Nutritionally speaking, they not only provide energy, but also supply significant amounts of minerals, B vitamins, protein, and fiber. Complex carbohydrate foods include beans, peas, nuts, seeds, vegetables, and whole-grain breads, cereals, and pasta. Starches, the best form of carbohydrates, include whole grains like brown rice, millet, buckwheat (also known as kasha), and barley, along with beans and root-like vegetables, such as potatoes, carrots, and yams. As you begin to use the herbal weight-management system you will want to add an increasing variety of unrefined complex carbohydrates. Remember that we are speaking of whole foods here. Refined carbohydrate foods such as white and brown sugar and white bread, crackers, most prepared cereals, pasta, and other foods made from white flour provide starch and calories but little else in the way of nutrients.

Carbohydrates:

1. Provide glucose for nerve tissues
2. Provide a primary source of energy

Attitude and Behavior Patterns

No matter how good your intentions are when you begin your weight-loss program, more likely than not, you will falter if you do not have the proper attitude. The key struggle for most people on any weight-loss program is remaining motivated. Emotionally speaking, most of us want every result instantly. This creates unrealistic expectations of how rapidly the process is going to take place.

The key to effective weight management is a common sense merging of the ancient and the modern. If you were to read every herb or nutritionally based weight-loss book ever written, you would find the same four fundamentals threading through them all. These variables integrate spiritual awareness, attitude, food choices, and preparation. If you combine them with the most recent herbal, nutritional, and dietary research, you will surely achieve success. Other important factors include:

Gratitude for the Grace of Food—whatever your religious or spiritual beliefs, it is essential that you both acknowledge and give thanks for the food you are about to eat. You may do this as a formal prayer, a moment of silence, the saying of grace, or performing some ritual or ceremony from your culture or faith. The key here is to create a conscious relationship between your desire to eat and the sustenance that food provides. Keep the following thought in mind as you get ready to learn more about herbal weight loss.

Herbs from the sea: Sea vegetables are popular in many weight-management programs because they have been found by some to stimulate a sluggish thyroid and may also reduce constipation that some people experience on high-protein, low-carbohydrate diets. By adding plenty of sea vegetables to the diet (nori, hijiki, dulse kombu, wakame), many people claim to have lost weight, gained energy, and obtained regular bowel movements.

A Creative Sense for How Food Comes to Us—the food on your plate, or in your hand, is about to reach the end of a long journey that began before recorded history. Through its relationship with societal changes, combined with the environment, science, music, art, history, and culture, your food has made a journey to become the recently planted seed that produced the tree, fruit, leaves, or flowers that have created what you are about to eat.

Food Choice and Preparation—unless you are eating fruit fresh off of the tree, all food, even the rawest or fastest of fast foods, must be prepared. When you can intelligently select, combine, cut, boil, bake, steam, microwave, pickle, ferment, freeze, or store a food, the process of fat reduction becomes all that much easier. Stop thinking about calories and begin to expand your choices. Use herbs in the preparation of fruit, vegetable, nut, seed, dairy, and grain food recipes. Try new types of vegetables such as those from the sea. As for sweeteners, toss the artificial sweeteners and go herbal. There are a wonderful array of herb-based sweeteners like Stevia, barley malt, 100 percent maple syrup, and more.

Protein, Fats, and Carbohydrates

Protein is essential to good health, but it seems of late that we have again become obsessed with high-protein diets. This is a yo-yo pattern that began at the end of World War II and has swung back and forth every few years since then. There was even a point

Eating—you must learn how to eat all over again, as if you were a baby. The art of eating must become a spiritual practice. If you eat on the run, unconsciously, then you will choose foods unconsciously as well. In the end you will keep the fat on and not have any idea how or why.

1. The first step to reducing stored body fat is to create the appropriate environment. If you are eating at home use beautiful silverware and a plate that you especially enjoy eating on. Pick a lovely drinking glass. My favorite is a cobalt blue champagne glass in a shiny brass stand. Play your favorite music. Remember to begin the meal with a few minutes of gratitude and contemplation.

2. The second step in conscious eating is to chew your food thoroughly. Through the chewing process both you and the food are transformed. You get to experience the full range of textures, tastes, and aromas. You are more easily fulfilled with less food intake as hundreds of neurological signals go off, enzymes are produced, and digestion is readied.

Herbs, Nutrition, and Healing—the art and science of reducing stored fat is learned. You must make a study based on the available knowledge. Each herb may affect the nervous system, the chakras, the organs, metabolism, and the emotions differently. It is important that you structure your eating program so that it will be lower in total fat, cholesterol, and saturated fat, while at the same time reducing your caloric intake and using herbs that will facilitate this process. The easiest way of doing this without great thought or discipline is to remove red meat from your diet and replace whole milk with part-skim milk or plant-based milk like soy, rice, or potato-based milk substitutes.

Certain herbs and green foods such as alfalfa, soy, and ginseng root have been found to have cholesterol-lowering properties. These valuable attributes are probably due to substances they contain known as saponins. As you begin to know your body better, and your emotional needs, you will develop a greater wisdom concerning what you eat it, how you eat it, and the lifestyle you surround these eating patterns with.

Carbohydrate Foods to Use:

Peas

Nuts

Vegetables

Whole Grains and whole-grain products including: seeds, brown
    rice, millet, buckwheat (kasha), barley

Potatoes

Yams

Carbohydrates to Avoid:

Refined or bleached white flour products found in many
    processed foods

Cookies

Cakes

Breads

Crackers

Semolina pasta products

Breakfast cereals

White rice

White sugar

in the late 1970s where some nutritionists were recommending a protein intake as high as 150 grams a day. People had to eat large amounts of red meat or drink all types of liquid proteins to achieve this level.

Many researches hold the more commonly accepted view that people can live healthily with a protein intake as low as thirty grams per day. Though this daily protein intake may be too low for most people, it is notable in its contrast to the high protein levels that were recommended by physicians not so long ago. Generally speaking, most healthy people will need approximately fifty to eighty grams of protein per day. In place of all that red meat and animal protein, we now know that combinations of various vegetarian foods are a much healthier choice.

Due to general lifestyle factors and the neverending attempt to find a magic way to lose weight, many of us have been led to believe that beef, chicken, whole-milk products, and eggs are the best sources of protein. In the 1980s, the focus returned again to reducing our fat intake by cutting back on red meat. We learned that although beef, chicken, whole-milk products, and eggs all had plenty of protein, they may also be laden with pesticides, hormones, saturated fats, and various body-polluting substances. Now it seems that the pendulum has swung the other way and people are reducing carbohydrates and increasing their intake of high-fat and high-protein foods. Luckily there are many foods that, when eaten alone or in combination with each other, offer quality protein without fat or undesirable chemicals.

Recent books on weight loss have shifted perspectives on the relationship of proteins, fats, and carbohydrates to weight control. There are mixed opinions on the accuracy of these new books. It is virtually impossible to discuss this issue without discussing the Atkins Diet.

The Atkins Program

Created by Robert Atkins, M.D., this diet program is based on the basic theory that dietary intake of almost all carbohydrates, but especially refined sugars and starches, abnormally increases production of insulin by the pancreas. This insulin increase results in increased fat storage and has a harmful effect on cardiovascular function. At the most extreme level, the additional insulin may result in insulin resistance. In this situation, cells do not respond to the efforts of insulin to deliver glucose. This in turn may lead to adult-onset diabetes. What both proponents and opponents of this diet agree upon is that after forty-eight hours on a very low carbohydrate diet, the body depletes its reserves of stored carbohydrates, known as glycogen, and begins to burn fat for fuel. Mainstream diet and nutrition experts see this change as unhealthy, but Atkins and his supporters say that there are no scientific studies to support this criticism.

Dr. Atkins may be accurate in theory, but in practice his diet is not the best choice available in my opinion. In replacing bread, pasta, and most sweet foods with high-fat foods like beef, cheese, and eggs, you may lose weight in the short run, but in the long run the saturated fat content will create problems for you. If you are someone with weight around your middle and any condition involving insulin resistance such as high serum triglycerides and low HDL (good cholesterol), a modified version of this diet may be of some value. If you do attempt this diet, I advise avoiding the high-fat meals that Dr. Atkins recommends and ask you to remember to keep your fat intake below 30 percent of your daily calories. Pay attention to keeping your saturated fat intake low by avoiding meat, butter, cream, and cheese.

Unfortunately, many animal foods contain pesticide residues, undesirable chemical additives, and hormones that are used in their production. If you want to use the high-protein approach to weight loss, shift your diet to include new types of high-quality protein, and decrease your intake of meats and high-fat dairy products. If you feel that you have to have some animal protein in your diet, then eat organically grown poultry and lamb or veal instead of beef or pork. If you are ready to make a greater adjustment to your diet, consider using low-fat milk products and grain and bean combinations as your primary protein sources. For example, you could include some healthy carbohydrates in the form of starchy vegetables, whole-wheat pasta, and fiber-rich 100 percent whole-grain bread.

Don't worry about losing the weight fast. A balanced diet with herbal support will result in a balanced, consistent weight loss. The faster you lose the weight, the more likely you are to gain it back. The key to remember is that excess caloric intake and sluggish metabolism will cause you to put on weight. It is still easier to

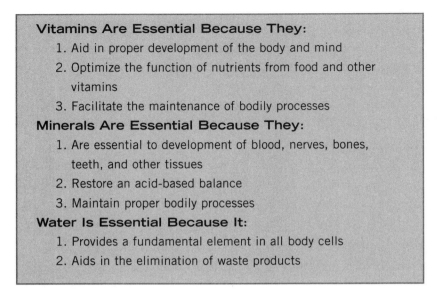

Vitamins Are Essential Because They:
1. Aid in proper development of the body and mind
2. Optimize the function of nutrients from food and other vitamins
3. Facilitate the maintenance of bodily processes

Minerals Are Essential Because They:
1. Are essential to development of blood, nerves, bones, teeth, and other tissues
2. Restore an acid-based balance
3. Maintain proper bodily processes

Water Is Essential Because It:
1. Provides a fundamental element in all body cells
2. Aids in the elimination of waste products

lose weight when you increase metabolism through herbs and then build a diet based on fruits, vegetables, grains, beans, and low-fat foods, including dairy products.

Five Winning Principles for Herbal Weight Loss

Principle #1: Break the fat storage cycle by making the right food choices and by practicing proper "food combining."

Fat is a concentrated source of calories with about twice as many calories (nine per gram) than are found in either carbohydrates or proteins. Fat-heavy meals also lack fiber, so you can eat hundreds of calories and never feel full. Even worse yet, when fat is eaten at the same time as simple carbohydrates, stored fat increases, blood fat levels rise, and the body's basic blood-sugar control mechanism is damaged. This "destructive" marriage of fats with carbohydrates actually slows down your metabolism and causes you to gain weight.

To begin your herbal weight-management program you must reduce your intake of all refined sugars and simple carbohydrates, especially avoiding the fat/carbohydrate combinations found in fried foods, cakes, cookies, sweet rolls, candy bars, and so on.

Expand your intake of whole grains, beans, lean proteins, and steamed or lightly grilled fresh vegetables. Season these foods with herbs to increase the range of flavors and textures and to reduce your desire for fats.

An effective approach to proper food combining is through a modified zone-style diet.

The Zone Diet

The Zone Diet was created by Dr. Barry Sears. The fundamental theory behind the Zone Diet is similar to that which Dr. Atkins uses to support his diet program: insulin production is greatly influenced by diet. The Zone Diet is less rigid in its point of view than the Atkins program in that Dr. Sears is more interested in creating an effective balance between carbohydrate, protein, and fat intake rather than restricting any one nutrient completely. According to this theory the balance between these three essential nutrients—carbohydrates 40 percent, proteins 30 percent, and fats 30 percent—supports the body in producing optimal levels of insulin. With insulin at a stable level, what Dr. Sears calls "a therapeutic zone"—neither rising nor dropping too quickly—the dieter can avoid the most common negative side effects of excessive insulin: chronic fatigue and constant weight gain. Be careful of your protein food choices, though. Many protein foods contain excess fat (most meats, eggs, whole milk). Moreover, some unbalanced protein/carbohydrate combinations may reduce the body's ability to release human growth hormone (HGH), a major fat-burning hormone.

The Zone Diet, when applied with a combination of thermogenic herbs and whole, unrefined foods (consisting primarily of vegetables, grains, beans, and low-fat dairy products), will guarantee that the body receives the proper ratio of the required amounts of low-fat protein at each meal, as well as a rich supply of essential fatty acids and fiber-rich fruits and vegetables. This will help the dieter maintain insulin levels within a therapeutic zone and assist in utilizing excess body fat, thus helping to lose weight.

Siberian Ginseng (Eleuthero—Eleutherococcus senticosus, Acanthopanax senticosus): Native to the Siberian Taiga region (northern China, southeastern Russia, Korea, and Japan), Siberian ginseng is known as *ci wu jia* in traditional Chinese medicine. Cultivated for its root and rhizomes, this herb is actually not a form of ginseng (genus Panax), but is a distant relative called Siberian ginseng because it is native to parts of China and Russia. Siberian ginseng has long held an esteemed place in traditional Chinese medicine, where it has been the most well known of the adaptogen herbs (adaptogens are agents that increase resistance to stress, fatigue, and disease by building up our general vitality and strengthening our normal body functions). The most profound changes that adaptogens help bring about are in the body's internal environment, especially in body temperature changes, diet, and exercise. Since these areas are what are most affected when a person is on a weight-loss program, this herb is particularly appropriate. Siberian ginseng works through the adrenal glands and helps support general mental and physical balance.

There are many vitamins, amino acids, and other principles found in Siberian ginseng, but the most important substances in this herb seem to be six glycosides called eleutherosides. It is difficult to dissociate the many components of the herb from the overall actions that are produced by it. It has a non-specific stimulant action on a physical and intellectual capacity that is free of the negative properties associated with other herbal stimulants. The stimulating action is reinforced by a protective action against various outside stresses including hard labor, chemical stress, and adrenal gland fatigue. The herb also enhances alertness, perception, and increases metabolism.

For many years, Soviet Olympic athletes have used this herb in their training regimens to promote stamina. As a result of their success, many nutritionists began to see the value of Siberian ginseng as part of an herbal weight-management program. This interest derives partly from the ability of the herb to improve the uptake of oxygen during exercise and increase general energy and vitality. This will assist the dieter in building endurance and recovering from workouts more readily.

Studies have demonstrated that Siberian ginseng offers a protective function when used with potentially toxic chemicals such as sodium barbital, ethanol, tetanus toxoid, and the chemotherapeutic agents used to treat cancer.

In Russia, it was originally used to reduce susceptibility to infections, but in recent years it has been used to help the body recover from stress and to improve mental clarity. It has also been used by cancer victims to lessen the side effects of chemotherapy and radiation treatments.

Eleuthero, as a fluid extract, possesses many healing and purifying properties, including:

1. Protects the body against stress, various chemical toxins, and environmental pollutants
2. Can be used therapeutically in conditions of acute and chronic radiation sickness, such as hemorrhaging, severe anemia, dizziness, nausea, vomiting, and headaches due to X rays (If you are receiving X rays or radiation treatments, use Eleuthero extract.)
3. Neutralizes the ill effects caused by drugs and other substances
4. Counteracts some of the side effects of cortisone treatments, such as adverse changes in the weight of the adrenals
5. Significantly improves human immune response
6. Prevents harmful effects of stress, such as stomach bleeding and disrupted production of adrenaline
7. Aids in the absorption and retention of some important protective nutrients, including vitamins Bl, B2, and C
8. May be valuable in the treatment of other long-term immune system dysfunction such as AIDS and chronic fatigue syndrome

> There is no combination of herbs and foods more protective against radiation and environmental pollutants than Siberian ginseng and sea vegetables.

Principle #2: Turn on your metabolism herbally and burn stored fat with the proper food choices and herbs.

Some foods burn "hotter" than others, i.e., they cause your body to expend more calories for heat, encourage activity, and are not as readily stored. Proteins and complex carbohydrates are "hot" burners. They are not as easily stored as fat and they tell your body it has plenty of fuel. This is part of the "thermic" or heat-producing effect of eating a high-protein or high-complex-carbohydrate meal, and it "turns on" your metabolism.

Combine lean vegetarian proteins, tofu, tempeh, and grains and beans (or fish, skinless chicken, lean beef, or lamb if you are not a vegetarian), with a variety of non-starch vegetables for especially energizing meals. If a meal does not contain concentrated carbohydrates (breads, grains, potatoes, etc.), you need not be particularly concerned about its fat content. Combine complex carbohydrates (grains and beans) with vegetables (and perhaps a small amount of lean protein) for tasty and filling meals.

Principle #3: Exercise to increase your metabolic efficiency and train your body to burn stored fat for energy.

Though this book is primarily concerned with herbs and weight management, it is impossible to discuss this subject without talking about exercise.

Exercise burns calories, and the greatest benefit comes after the exercise has ended. If you walk briskly for a mere thirty minutes per day, you will increase your calorie burning for the rest of the entire twenty-four-hour period. Adding a moderate amount of upper body exercise or weight lifting will improve your energy expenditure even more by adding calorie-burning lean muscle tissue to your body.

Cuwijia: This herb is used in Chinese medicine to combat fatigue and enhance immune activity, but Chinese researchers also note that the herb increases the burning of fat during strenuous exercise. It shifts the energy source that fuels exercise from muscle carbohydrate to fat, and it slows down the buildup of the lactic acid that always accompanies exercise and leads to muscle burnout and fatigue. The data also suggests that the product can increase exercise endurance and lean body mass (muscle without the fat).

For weight loss, plan on walking briskly for at least thirty minutes every day. This is the best done either before or after breakfast. A walk early in the day while the body's temperature is still rising will invigorate you. A second time to walk is after your last meal of the day. Walking after meals is a particularly good practice for diabetics and for those genetically prone to developing diabetes.

An effective exercise program can be as basic or complex as you wish. It all depends on you. Its consistency and regularity are the defining factors in your success. Many people who are in too much of a hurry to lose weight are also too eager to exercise without using common sense. When developing your exercise program it is important that you remember the following:

1. Make sure that you pick the appropriate exercise regime for you. Don't do what someone else does without thinking it out first.
2. Once you have designed your program, perform your exercises correctly.
3. Take your time. Working out vigorously without attention to the movement is a prescription for injury.

Remember: Begin any exercise by warming up slowly. Non-weight-bearing, range-of-motion exercise will bring more blood to your muscles while slowly increasing your heart rate. After doing the non-weight-bearing movements, then you may gently

> **Kelp (Fucus vesiculosis):** Also known as Bladderwrack, kelp is a sea vegetable that is a well-researched thyroid tonic containing significant amounts of iodine as well as vitamins and mineral salts including potassium, magnesium, calcium, and iron.
>
> Iodine is crucial to the maintenance of a healthy thyroid. As a source of iodine, kelp assists in making thyroid hormones, which are necessary for the maintenance of normal metabolism in all cells of the body.
>
> Kelp increases the body's ability to burn fat during exercise. It also contains nutrients that promote the health of various organs. The mucilage in Bladderwrack has an appetite suppressive function and because of this, it is included as an ingredient in many commercial weight-loss formulas. The totality of the elements it contains can have a favorable effect in activating and stimulating certain endocrine glands, osmotic exchanges, and the elimination of waste materials.

stretch to increase muscle flexibility and reduce the chance of injury. Absolutely avoid bouncing or ballistic movements during this exercise since this can lead to injury.

As you lose weight, your center of gravity will shift. For this reason, it is important that you strengthen both your back and abdominal muscles. When doing abdominal strengthening exercises, it is essential that you keep your knees bent.

Avoid:

- Deep knee-bends and toe-touches when your legs are locked (straight)
- Jogging or running on hard surfaces
- Forcing yourself beyond what is comfortable

Principle #4: Add fiber to your diet.

The best choice in dietary fiber comes in the form of lightly cooked green vegetables and high-fiber herbs. Avoid refined and processed foods whenever possible.

What exactly is dietary fiber? Quite simply, dietary fiber is derived from the portion of a plant that has not been digested by enzymes in the intestinal tract.

Fiber is an essential element of any healthy diet and effective weight-control program. Hot and cold breakfast cereals (especially those with added psyllium seed husks), noodles, pasta, and various whole grains, including breads and especially brown rice, will give you many of the essential nutrients you require while reducing fat intake and still giving you a sense of fullness. Fiber slows down food consumption so that your body has a chance to signal that you have eaten enough. It adds bulk to the meal to give you a feeling of satiation. It slows the increase in the blood sugar level that follows any meal. Fiber carries waste products from the body and, especially if it comes from lightly cooked vegetables, supplies important minerals and antioxidants.

As in every other aspect of this program, it is essential that you avoid going to extremes. Many people will use large amounts of bran, especially wheat bran, to speed up weight loss. The problem here is that bran and bran-rich foods contain naturally occurring substances called phytates. Proper levels of various minerals such as calcium, iron, zinc, magnesium, and phosphorous are essential to good health and effective weight loss. Phytates can reduce the absorption of these minerals in the intestinal tract. Vary your fiber sources. Avoid too much scratchy wheat bran, but eat grains, such as oats and barley, and starchy vegetables, such as sweet potatoes and yams (without adding butter and sugar). Try to eliminate all canned and frozen foods, as these often contain hidden fats and sugars.

The key then is to avoid mono-diets, or diets where large amounts of any one food dominates. If your diet is varied, then phytates do not pose a problem.

Some herbal sources of fiber include psyllium seed husks and the use of the clear sea vegetable derivative agar-agar in preparing low-calorie desserts and custards.

Principle #5: Use anti-fat nutrients and herbal thermogenic enhancers.

Many individuals who are overweight find that they need a little help to jump-start their ability to burn fat. Certain herbs can promote thermogenesis, which occurs in brown adipose tissue and reverses the body's tendency to store fat by increasing the production of heat-energy, which burns calories.

One of the chief drawbacks of calorie-restricted diets is their tendency to lower the body's rate of energy production. Ma huang, with its active ingredient, ephedrine, is the most effective thermogenic. Many herbal weight-loss products contain ma huang in large doses. However, the consumption of ma huang can result in unwanted side effects. Pregnant women, diabetics, and people with serious hypertension should not use thermogenesis.

Thermogenic Enhancers

Many ephedra-based formulas also contain the herb guarana. Guarana is the base ingredient of various popular soda and tea beverages in South America. It is named after the tribe it was commonly associated with, the Guaranis, who used it as a means to increase stamina and endurance. The guarana used in weight-loss formulas is made from the crushed seeds of a caffeine-rich South American shrub.

Used alone, guarana has a caffeine content similar to coffee and is found in many thermogenically based weight-loss formulas. The herb works by speeding up metabolism and burning fat. Unfortunately, this is an herb that is easily abused. When combined with ephedra, it makes the stimulant effect more powerful and even dangerous. There are reports that when used improperly or in high doses this combination may cause high blood pressure, stroke, or even death. Many professional herbalists avoid using it.

However, there are a number of herbs that increase metabolism thermogenically without any negative effects. Among these are the seaweed known as kelp, which activates the thyroid gland

Mustard Seeds: Used since ancient times as a medicine, mustard seeds are often used in healing poultices. As a cooking spice, black mustard seeds are essential ingredients in Indian dishes. The more common yellow mustard seeds are used in pickling vegetables and in making relishes, curries, and salads. The type of mustard that is spread on sandwiches comes from ground mustard seeds. In addition to all this, it is a spice that should be used liberally because of its thermogenic quality.

as well as mustard seed and cayenne pepper. The latter of these two will help start the thermogenic process and make other substances, including caffeine and ephedrine, more effective as thermogenic aids. This may help a person who intends to use these last two herbs in smaller amounts.

Like most supplements, thermogenics should be taken within a half-hour of meals. This is especially true if you experience nervousness or jitteriness. To minimize impact, the thermogenic program should be started in the morning and completed by 3 P.M., as taking it after 3 P.M. may result in difficulty sleeping. For the same reason, thermogenics should not be used with teas, colas, coffee, or other caffeinated beverages.

For persons trying to stop smoking, thermogenics can help prevent weight gain, since nicotine itself is a mild thermogenic agent. When people quit smoking this removal of a thermogenic agent may contribute to a slight weight gain, especially when combined with an increase in the consumption of sweets.

The daily consumption of products containing ephedrine and caffeine in conjunction with aspirin, or their natural equivalents, has been shown to increase thermogenesis also. However, this type of treatment is considered unsafe by many doctors and herbalists. Thermogenesis can be positively affected by green tea and the following major thermogenic herbs: kola nut, gooroo nut, yerba maté, guarana, iodine from fucus, white willow bark, and cayenne. Kola nuts are known to strengthen the heart and boost energy and

> **Cayenne (Capsicum frutescens):** Native to tropical America, cayenne is a perennial in the wild. The fruit of the cayenne plant is used as an appetizer, digestive, and stimulant. It lowers blood cholesterol and prevents the rise in cholesterol levels that usually follows the ingestion of foods high in cholesterol. Used as a stimulant, cayenne has been recommended in weight-loss programs with a thermogenic tilt. It stimulates the production of ATP (fuel), thus increasing thermogenesis and stimulating the cells so more calories are burned. It also increases glucose metabolism, lowers blood serum triglyceride concentration, and stimulates the release of adrenaline from the adrenal medulla and the sympathetic nervous system. Capsaicin, the pungent element in cayenne, elevates the mitochondria's ability to efficiently use oxygen, and raises the metabolic resting rate.

alertness. White willow bark contains salicin, which the body converts to salicylic acid, which helps the blood flow more freely.

Nutrients that can impact the thermogenesis process are pantothenic acid, essential fatty acids, vitamin B6, vitamin C, ginger root, zinc, manganese, magnesium, and niacin.

Nine More Tips on Losing Weight Easily and Efficiently

1. Adopt a vegetarian diet. Vegetarian diets are naturally low in fat and calories and high in fiber.
2. Drink at least eight glasses of fluids every day. Water, fresh vegetable juice, herbal tea, or vegetable broth is best. This will give you a feeling of fullness and at the same time cleanse your body of toxic substances that accumulate as you burn fat. Do not drink a lot while you are eating, however.
3. Instead of eating three meals a day, divide your caloric intake between six very small meals. This will reduce the desire for between-meals snacking and will reduce the outpouring of insulin that accompanies large meals, which can contribute to the accumulation of fat.

Neroli (Citrus aurantium): This herbal agent is obtained by extraction of the freshly picked flowers of the bitter orange tree as well as citrus rinds of this tree harvested while still green. Most Citrus aurantium is produced in Italy, France, and on a smaller scale in Morocco, Cyprus, Haiti, Taiwan, and the Comores Islands. At its nutritional peak, Citrus aurantium is rich in flavonoids and contains an agent called synephrine, which like ephedrine, is an edregernic amine. Both of these agents may enhance metabolic rate, increase fat burning, and spare muscle protein. Research shows that Citrus aurantium increases the breakdown of stored fat (lipolysis) by increasing the activity of the BAT cells and thus thermogenesis and the metabolic rate. Unlike ephedra (ma huang), caffeine, or guarana, Citrus aurantium works without stimulating the central nervous system, and thus has none of the associated side effects or health risks.

Citrus aurantium is effective in an herbal weight-management program because, unlike ephedrine, the use of synephrine seldom produces any of the agitation associated with ephedrine use. In fact, synephrine may be even more thermogenic (increasing resting metabolic rate) than ephedrine while causing less stimulation to the heart rate and blood pressure than ephedrine. According to the most up-to-date research, synephrine is safe, with no serious side effects. It is for these reasons and others that bitter orange extract has been added to many herbal weight-loss formulas as a replacement for ephedra.

Citrus aurantium is also rich in flavonoids. Flavonoids are powerful antioxidants with anti-blood-clotting properties. Researchers have found that they can counter oxygen-caused damage in the body (such as fatty tissue deposits), can help avoid heart problems, and can promote better circulation and overall health as free radicals in the body are eliminated through their antioxidant effect.

4. Do not keep unhealthy snack foods in your house, even if it's to entertain friends. It's too tempting to help yourself to snacks. What you might do is prepare yourself several

baked potatoes and keep them in the refrigerator. Then, when you feel hungry, cut one in half and eat it with a tablespoon of yogurt.

5. Be moderate in your use of goitrogen-rich foods. According to the *Tufts University Diet & Nutrition Newsletter* (March 1985: 5), foods, such as raw cabbage, cauliflower, turnips, kale, rutabagas, Brussels sprouts, horseradish, and broccoli all contain substances known as goitrogens. When consumed in excess amounts, goitrogens can result in goiter, an iodine deficiency disease. This condition can result in enlargement of the thyroid gland and can also alter metabolism. If you have had difficulty losing weight in the past due to slow metabolism, you may wish to use these foods in moderation.

6. Exercise regularly.

7. Do not get into the habit of using food as an emotional reward.

8. Eat slowly and concentrate on what you're doing. Reading or watching TV while you eat will rob you of the consciousness of enjoying what you eat.

9. Drink herbal tea instead of soda or juice.

Remember: Ultimately the goal of any herbal weight-management program should have three parts:

1. Thermogenic fat burning
2. Antioxidant effect
3. Appetite suppression

   With these three factors working together synergistically, an herbal program can promote healthy, long-term weight loss.

Chapter 3

Losing Weight with Nutritional Body Detoxification

We live in a highly polluted environment, and what we don't see *can* hurt us. Even when we attempt to live a healthy lifestyle, we are bombarded by radioactivity, water and air pollutants, and chemicals and hidden fats in our food. Detoxification with herbs helps create a healthier environment for healthy weight management.

Plants are naturally cleansing and detoxifying for the body and mind. They help to neutralize the waste products of metabolism, purify the blood, and cleanse and help form tissue in the body. Because of these favorable effects, herbs and spices (especially in combination with juicing) are particularly effective in helping a person lose unwanted pounds and achieve their ideal weight.

Often an overlooked component in weight-loss programs, detoxification is critical if the program is to be a success. Based on a combination of ancient Chinese herbs and Western detoxifying formulas, this chapter provides powerful detoxification and cleansing actions. Herbal body purification helps to carry the released toxins safely out of the body.

Asian herbs such as glucomannan, platycodon, schizonepeta, atracytlodes, tang-kuei, and Chinese peony have historically been used to reduce water retention, promote water metabolism (flushing), inhibit cholesterol absorption, remove toxins through the skin and through the digestive and excretory systems, tone the skin and underlying tissues, promote healthy excretion, and promote lipid metabolism (fat burning).

Glucomannan: This is a calorie-free, high-fiber herb which is obtained from the root of the Amorphophallus Konjac plant. It has been used as a food in Asia for more than one thousand years. This pectin-like powder is usually taken in capsule form. Its value in weight-management programs results from the gel consistency it takes when wet. Glucomannan absorbs liquid up to fifty times its weight, giving the person who ingests it a feeling of fullness. Glucomannan helps to absorb toxic substances produced during digestion, and then eliminates them before they pass into the bloodstream.

Precautions: people with diabetes may have to decrease the dosage of medication, since glucomannan may improve glycemic control.

Glucomannan is effective for:
- Cleaning the digestive system
- Weight loss
- Cholesterol reduction
- Glucose reduction
- Bowel health

Easily assimilated organic minerals, particularly calcium, silicon, and potassium, found in herbs and spices, help restore mineral and biochemical balance in cells and tissues. Mineral imbalances lead to diminished oxygenation, a cause for the disease and premature aging of cells.

Herbs and spices are packed with vitamins, minerals, enzymes, natural sugars, and trace elements. (In juicing, almost 100 percent of the vital nutritive elements are directly assimilated into the bloodstream without putting a strain on the digestive system.)

Fresh herbs are extremely important for normalizing the acid-alkaline balance in the tissues and blood by providing an alkaline surplus. This is important because over-acidity is a contributing factor in disease development, and is present in most conditions of ill health.

Vitally important from a therapeutic point of view also are the various colors that herbs and vegetables come in—reds, greens, yellows, and even blues. These, in their variety of shades and intensities, influence digestive and assimilative processes, take part in the metabolism of proteins and cholesterol, and increase production of red blood corpuscles.

Radioactivity

Everything in our environment has some radioactivity. The water, food, soil, and our bodies all contain trace amounts of naturally occurring radioactive isotopes. Most of these background radioactive particles dissolve in water. Since more than 90 percent of the human body is made of water, it is natural for our bodies to contain these radioactive particles. Luckily, there is no long-term internal buildup of radioactive isotopes, since most of this radioactivity is quickly excreted. Smokers, however, are not so lucky. Tobacco contains trace levels of radioactivity, some of which don't wash out of the lungs. These radioactive particles accumulate there and bombard delicate lung tissue with low-level alpha radiation, the same kind of radiation emitted by plutonium.

Chemicals in Our Food

Every food and every herb is made up of acids, alkaloids, and nutrients—all chemicals. Coffee contains caffeine; yerba maté contains mateine; an orange is rich in ascorbic acid, inositol, biotin, tartaric acid, choline, nucleotides, and peroxidase. It is not chemicals per se that are the source of the problem. It is the source of the chemicals that is the problem. Nutritious foods whether prepared at home or purchased commercially have colors, flavors, and textures that are also nutritionally rich. That is because these colors, flavors, and textures come from a merging of different herbs, spices, aromatic oils, and food ingredients that make them not only tasteful but nutritionally rich as well.

On the other hand, we often choose foods manufactured in a laboratory rather than by Mother Nature. Many of the manufactured foods that have become a regular part of our eating patterns are nutritionally destitute, refined foods combined with synthetic additives used in processing and packaging to artificially preserve color and flavor. Other synthetic additives are added to create texture and aroma for what we eat. When you eat these foods, you are choosing highly processed, nutritionally depleted foods. These foods may look good, smell good, and taste good, but they really are nothing but a chemical feast. They create a toxic environment in the body.

Your body does not require, and cannot make use of, these additives. In fact, your detoxifying organs—liver, kidney, spleen, lungs, and skin—must neutralize and eliminate them from your body. This detoxification process depletes energy and creates a state of imbalance. When much of the food you eat is processed with these artificial ingredients, your body is not getting the nutritional energy it needs. In this diminished state, body polluting additives do not get eliminated and instead build to toxic levels. Eventually, this toxic overload may make you sick.

Non-organic meats and milk are laden with pesticides, antibiotics, hormones, unhealthy fats, and various other undesirable elements. And because we have polluted our oceans, the fish we eat are also full of toxins.

How Can We Reverse This Body Pollution?

A key element to any herbal weight-loss program is stimulation of various organs of detoxification and elimination. The organs in this process include the kidneys, the colon, and most importantly the liver. The liver plays several roles in detoxification: it filters the blood to remove large toxins, synthesizes and secretes bile full of cholesterol and other fat-soluble toxins, and disassembles unwanted chemicals with enzymes. The liver is also important in reducing the buildup of free radicals. Once the liver has modified a toxin, it needs to be eliminated from the body as soon as possible. One of the primary routes of elimination is through bile.

The first step in supporting proper liver function and bile flow is following a health-promoting diet low in animal foods and

Alpha Lipoic Acid: It is known as a universal antioxidant, since it is found in virtually every cell of the body, and because it counteracts excessive free radical activity via several mechanisms in cell membranes as well as inside cells.

Alpha lipoic acid is also a cofactor for some of the key enzymes (alpha keto acid dehydrogeneses) involved in generating energy from food and oxygen in mitochondria.

Alpha lipoic acid is helpful in controlling excess sugar levels by improving carbohydrate metabolism and ensuring that fewer carbohydrates (sugars) are converted into fats. This also improves energy levels, as the metabolized carbohydrates become energy for your mind and body.

sugar, and high in whole-plant foods such as vegetables, grains, legumes, fruits, nuts, and seeds. Such a diet will provide a wide range of essential nutrients the liver needs to carry on its important functions. There are many special foods rich in factors that help protect the liver from damage and improve liver function. Among these are garlic, legumes, and onions; good sources of water-soluble fibers such as pears, oat bran, apples, and legumes; cabbage family vegetables (especially broccoli); Brussels sprouts and cabbage; and artichokes, beets, carrots, dandelion, and many herbs and spices including milk thistle, turmeric, cinnamon, and licorice.

For this reason, it is important to develop dietary patterns that you can apply while using detoxifying herbs.

Here is a guide of what to eat and what to avoid while detoxifying and easing your body into a weight-loss mode.

Foods to Include/Foods to Avoid to Maximize Healthy Weight Loss

Baking Bread at Home

Allowed—Unleavened products, matzoh, natural yeast
Avoid—Baking soda, baking powder, preserved yeast

Beverages

Allowed—Herbal teas (chamomile, mint, papaya); grain-based coffee substitutes; fresh vegetable juice; hot chocolate soy milk; or rice beverages

Avoid—Fruit juice (too high on the glycemic index), alcohol, caffeine, hot chocolate, coffee, carbonated beverages, artificial fruit drinks

Alcohol

Allowed—Non-alcoholic beer; wine that has the alcohol removed

Avoid—Alcoholic beverages tend to be high in calories and low in other nutrients. Even moderate drinkers may need to drink less if they wish to achieve ideal health and maintain steady weight loss.

Heavy drinkers may lose their appetites for foods containing essential nutrients. Vitamins and mineral deficiencies occur commonly in heavy drinkers—in part because of poor intake, but also because alcohol alters the absorption and use of some essential nutrients. These sub-clinical nutritional deficiencies may cause a person to eat more high-calorie foods.

Sustained or excessive alcohol consumption by pregnant women has caused birth defects. Pregnant women should limit alcohol intake to two ounces or less on any single day.

Heavy drinking may also cause a variety of serious conditions such as cirrhosis of the liver and some neurological disorders. Cancer of the throat and neck is much more common in people who drink and smoke than in those people who don't.

Carbohydrates

Allowed—Foods based on whole-grain sources including: whole wheat, rye, corn, whole unrefined corn meal, barley, buckwheat (kasha), millet, and brown rice

Such foods might include 100 percent whole-grain breads, pita pockets, muffins, pasta, and pancake mixes.

Avoid—refined white flour products, such as white rice, white flour pita pockets, white bread, and other low-fiber wheat, rye,

and other dark breads that are made from white flour with coloring and preservatives added

Chocolate
Allowed—Carob and carob powders
Avoid—Milk chocolate and carob candy bars containing hydro-
genated or partially hydrogenated vegetable oil

Dairy Products
Allowed—Raw milk; sugar-free, low-fat yogurt; and buttermilk
Avoid—All processed and imitation butter (margarine); any
yogurts containing Nutrasweet, sugar, cane syrup, gelatin, modified food starch, or any artificial colors or flavors; high-fat cheeses
and any pasteurized processed cheeses or cheese spreads

Note: instead of cream cheese use Neufchatel cheese. When
choosing hard cheeses try dairy-free soy and rice-based cheese
substitutes. You can also make your own low-fat herbed spreads
with tofu-based cream cheese.

Desserts
Allowed—Fruit flavored yogurt, fresh fruit compote, or any
desserts listed in the Recipe Section in the back of the book
Avoid—Ice cream

Dressings
Allowed—Packaged, low-fat, herbal-based dressings that are free
of sugar and any artificial ingredients; herbed vinegar; tofu; non-
fat yogurt; extra-virgin olive oil; Tabasco sauce; homemade
ketchup; homemade barbecue sauce; natural mayonnaise (homemade or natural, eggless, tofu-based variety)
Avoid—Pourable salad dressing (read label for oil content and
composition; some may contain coconut or palm oil); commercially bottled or packaged dressings containing monosodium glu-
tamate (MSG), modified food starch, artificial colors, flavors, or
preservatives; ketchup with sugar; A1 sauce

Note: if a recipe calls for mayonnaise, choose low-fat yogurt, buttermilk, or a low-calorie eggless mayonnaise that is available in a health-food store.

Fruits
Allowed—Fresh fruit in moderation
Avoid—All dried, stewed, canned, and sweetened fruit

Nuts
Allowed—All fresh, raw nuts in moderation; nuts in the shell; blanched and home-roasted whole nuts
Avoid—Roasted, dry roasted, and/or salted nuts, especially peanuts

Fats and Oils
Allowed—Foods rich in monounsaturated fats, and in omega 3 and omega 6 fatty acids (flaxseed oil, pumpkin seed oil, soybean oil, extra-virgin olive oil, eggless mayonnaise, and olive oil)

Note: olive oil contains 70 to 85 percent unsaturated oleic acid and 9 to 14 percent unsaturated linoleic acid. In addition to its nutritional value (more than 85 percent unsaturated fatty acids), olive oil is often used to facilitate elimination of bile. For this purpose it is best taken in the morning on an empty stomach. Olive oil is also used in cases of moderate arterial hypertension.

Avoid—Sour cream and other whole milk or cream-based dairy products; highly processed and chemically refined fats and oils (unsaturated as well as saturated); margarine or any type of mayonnaise; hydrogenated and partially hardened vegetable shortenings; foods high in both saturated fats and cholesterol, such as lard, lard-based shortenings, beef fat, beef fat–based shortening, and butter; coconut oil; palm kernel oil; foods high in saturated fats, such as meat drippings

Read package labels when choosing processed foods. Remember that "vegetable oil" could mean coconut or palm oil, both high in saturated fat.

Note: remember which foods are dietary sources of saturated fats and cholesterol. As a rule of thumb, saturated fats and cholesterol are generally found in foods from animal sources, while polyunsaturated fats come from vegetable sources—coconut and palm oil are the exceptions.

Protein

Allowed—Combinations of grains and beans in various forms are the easiest way of getting balanced combinations of proteins and complex carbohydrates. Beans should be soaked overnight so that they will not require as much cooking. The best beans to work with are soybeans, garbanzo beans (chick peas), dried lentils, kidney beans, lima beans, and split peas. Beans form an even higher quality protein when combined with grains such as brown rice, millet, and corn or sesame seeds. There are many other excellent vegetarian proteins. These include:

1. Raw, unsalted nuts: almonds, pignolias, Brazil nuts, or pecans (Ground meal or butters of these nuts are also excellent, but should be raw and unsalted at all times.)
2. Tempeh
3. Sesame seeds or meal (Protein-aids brand is best)
4. Green magma
5. Brewer's yeast (I recommend brands that are calcium-magnesium balanced.)
6. Sunflower seeds or meal, raw, unsalted
7. Tofu
8. Micro-algae (spirulina, chlorella, etc.)

If you are not presently leaning toward a vegetarian diet, avoid meat, eggs, and high-fat dairy products. Use some fish and poultry when you feel the urge.

Herbs, Spices, and Seasonings

Allowed—All herbs, especially cumin, sage, tarragon, thyme, coriander, garlic, onion, parsley, marjoram, mustard, cayenne pepper, salt-reduced soy sauce, pure sugar-free herb extracts

Choose low-sodium seasonings such as lemon or lime juice, herbs, salt substitutes (check with medical adviser before using). Use fresh ground black and white pepper. Both have a thermogenic effect.

Avoid—Salt; chemical imitation flavor; barbecue or high-sodium spices including soy sauce with any sugar, preservatives, artificial flavors, or colors added; high-sodium condiments such as ketchup, relish, soy sauce, or barbecue sauce; prepared frozen dinners; processed or salted meats, fish, and poultry; potato chips, pretzels, salted nuts, and salted, buttered popcorn; canned vegetables, canned soups; and powdered bouillon

Note: if you have high blood pressure, it is important to avoid hidden sodium in foods. Choose salt-free bakery goods, unsalted nuts, unsalted unbuttered popcorn, unsalted fresh or frozen vegetables, and homemade soups.

Soups

Allowed—Homemade soup (e.g., salt-free, vegetable), natural vegetable bouillon from a health-food store (Use arrowroot starch to thicken soups and as a replacement for cream.)

Avoid—Canned and creamed soups (thickened, commercial bouillon, fat stock)

Sweets

Allowed—Carob powder, barley malt, or rice syrup (In recipes use small amounts of maple syrup or honey.)

Avoid—Foods containing molasses, refined sugars (white, brown, turbinado), anything but 100 percent pure maple syrup, and dehydrated raw sugar cane juice, candy, syrups, high-fructose corn syrup, glucose, eating sweets between meals

Note: though sweeteners such as honey and maple syrup are acceptable in a natural food diet they are too high on the glycemic index and can create pancreatic stress which may lead to yo-yo dieting.

When buying packaged foods, read the labels for information

on sugar content. I cannot stress strongly enough the importance of avoiding too much concentrated sugar. Research has shown refined white sugar to be a source of food sensitivity, particularly low blood sugar (hypoglycemia), and elevation of triglyceride levels, which could result in hypertension as well as a loss of minerals, including calcium from the body.

When discussing sugar, most people think of table sugar (sucrose), but there are many other types of refined sugar as well. Being familiar with all the other labels for sugar will be of help when you're grocery shopping. They are glucose (dextrose), high fructose corn sweetener, maltose, and lactose. Limit sugary desserts. Instead, top off your meal occasionally with fresh fruits, which both satisfy your desire for sweets and provide valuable nutrients.

To reduce sugar intake from soft drinks, limit intake or dilute them with seltzer water.

If you add sugar to foods such as coffee, tea, or cereal, add less each time; you may gradually eliminate it.

Vegetables

Allowed—Vegetables in season; all raw and not overcooked fresh or frozen vegetables; root vegetables; beans
Avoid—Canned vegetables and fried potatoes in any form

Water

Allowed—Steamed, distilled water; osmotically filtered water; some bottled spring waters
Avoid—Tap water, especially if fluoridated (If not fluoridated, boil before using and run through a water filtration unit.)

Note: water is as important as any essential nutrient. Water is especially valuable for body detoxification and weight management because it can:

1. Suppress the appetite naturally and help the body
   metabolize stored fat. By drinking water and correcting
   fluid retention, more fat is used as fuel. This is because the
   liver is free to metabolize fat at top speed.

> **Water:** An overweight person needs more water than a thin person does since larger people have larger metabolic loads. Since we know that water is the key to fat metabolism, drinking water is essential to weight loss and maintaining good health during the stress of dieting.
>
> Dieters should keep in mind that they normally receive a large portion of their daily water needs through their food, which can be 70 to 90 percent water. During dieting, the food intake is reduced and as a result, the person is not getting their normal supply of water, let alone the extra water they need to flush out the metabolic by-products. This results in a "hidden hunger" in dieters as the body is craving food—not for its calorie content, but for its water content.

2. Increase kidney function. When the kidneys don't work to capacity, some of their load is dumped on the liver, forcing it to metabolize less fat.
3. Help to wash out by-products of metabolism.
4. Prevent accumulation of body (and drug) toxins.
5. Help in maintaining all normal body functions, such as temperature control and electrolyte balance, and prevent constipation. Ample water is also important in preventing sagging skin during fat loss.
6. Keep the skin healthy. If the body can't get rid of the by-products from metabolizing stored body fat via kidney excretion, the skin is called upon to help excrete these by-products. People often overlook the role of the skin in excreting toxins and the role of water in having healthy skin.

Reducing Radioactive Toxicity with Herbs

As you design your herbal weight-management program, keep in mind that there are also herbs that are effective at cleansing the system of toxic metals and metabolic and other undesirables. The ingredients listed below are all available at your local health food or natural food store in tablet, capsule, or liquid forms. If available in powder or liquid form they may be taken by placing them in a blender filled with fresh apple or papaya juice or, if you wish, ginger or red-clover tea. Use them according to the directions.

Bee pollen, nutritional yeast, and chlorella (a type of micro algae): These are rich in nucleic acids, an important group of organic substances found especially in the nuclei of all living cells. Nucleic acids are essential to life, and two of the most important nucleic acids, ribonucleic acid (RNA) and deoxyribonucleic acid (DNA), are crucial to the transmission of hereditary patterns.

Pectin: Powerful detoxifying qualities, lowers cholesterol

Papaya enzyme: Helps digest some of the waste matter that may remain in the stomach

Sodium alginate: Absorbs toxins

Psyllium seed: Increases bile acid secretion and supplies bulk

Liquid chlorophyll: Increases mineral absorption and helps to reestablish health-building bacteria in the system

Beet-root powder: Helps loosen the mucous buildup from the colon walls

Bentonite: A natural clay that is well known among healers for its ability to absorb toxins

Flaxseed: High fiber and healing to the colon

The Role of the Liver and Lipotropics in Detoxification

The liver acts in the digestive process by excreting bile, which helps with digestion and the absorption of fats. By breaking fat down into miniscule drops, which are easily digested, bile acts as a buffer for the intestinal contents. When bile is combined with fatty acid, the acids become water soluble and easier to absorb.

The liver is the primary site of lipotropic action. By definition, lipotropics are nutritional factors that serve to prevent the accumulation of fat in the liver, and they usually aid in the detoxification of metabolic wastes and other toxins. Some lipotropics help to emulsify fats so that the blood can more readily transport them. Other lipotropics work more directly with the digestion, either by

Milk thistle (Silybum marianum): A member of the sunflower family, milk thistle has purple flowers and milky white leaf veins. The medicinal use of milk thistle can be traced back to ancient Greece and Rome. This herb is a valuable component of any herbal purification program. Today researchers around the world have completed more than three hundred scientific studies that attest to the benefits of this herb, particularly in detoxification of the liver.

A group of flavonoid compounds found in milk thistle seems to exert a tremendous effect on protecting the liver from damage as well as enhancing detoxification processes by acting as a powerful antioxidant. One of the key manners is by preventing the depletion of glutathione. The level of glutathione in the liver is directly connected to the liver's ability to detoxify. When the glutathione content is higher, the liver has a greater capacity to detoxify harmful chemicals. Silybum marianum not only prevents the depletion of glutathione, it also increases the level of glutathione of the liver by up to 35 percent.

Silybum marianum has been shown to have benefits that include:

1. Treating liver diseases of various types including cirrhosis; chronic hepatitis; fatty infiltration of the liver (chemical- and alcohol-induced fatty liver); and inflammation of the bile duct
2. Aiding in the treatment and prevention of gallstones
3. Protecting the liver from toxins, including drugs, poisons, and chemicals
4. Helping to clear psoriasis

stimulating the liver to produce bile, which is then sent to the gallbladder, or by stimulating the gallbladder to release its stored bile into the digestive tract to help emulsify fats.

Herbal lipotropics include dandelion root, barberry, bearberry, Oregon grape root, turmeric, milk thistle, wall germander, and many others. Several herbal lipotropics, including bearberry and turmeric, also act as insulin potentiators.

Some people report a reduction of fat and cellulite from the use of lipotropics; however, the biochemical explanations for such reports at this point are largely theoretical.

Milk and Milk Products

The addition of dairy products will increase your protein quotient up from adequate to high. If you choose low-fat milk products over full-fat milk products, you will reduce the saturated fat you eat as well. Unfortunately, many people do not handle milk products well or have allergic reactions to them. The solution to this problem is to increase your intake of plant-based milk substitutes.

Plant-Based Milk Substitutes

Soy Milk: Back in the late 1960s when I began my own interest in herbs and holistic health, soy milk was a revelation for many people who wanted to avoid dairy products. Of course, soy has limitations of its own. Though I find it as desirable as cow's milk, two of the nutritional limitations of soy milk are:

1. It is low in the calcium, vitamin A, and vitamin D found in cow, sheep, or goat milk. The solution now is that there are a number of products available in health-food stores that are fortified with these nutrients.
2. Many people, as they do with cow milk, have allergic or sensitivity reactions to soy.

Potato-Based Milk Substitute: It may not sound all that exciting, but potato-based milk substitutes are great. Most have as much as 60 percent less fat than most soy milks and are free of hydrogenated oils. These products usually come in a powdered form that easily mixes with water. They are also rich in calcium.

Grain- and Nut-Based Milk Substitutes: There are many different non-dairy, milk-like beverages found around the world. Horchata is a traditional Mexican-based rice beverage that you can find in Mexican restaurants. Amazake, a thick beverage, has been popular in Japan for hundreds of years, and is very popular among health-food store customers in the United States. Amazake is prepared from brown rice that has been cooked, mixed with a special rice culture (koji) or special enzymes, and then incubated for six to ten hours. During this incubation period, the complex starches in the rice are broken down into sugars that are more easily digested. Amazake may have different flavors such as almond or carob added.

In the last few years many companies have begun producing a "rice-milk" product. This is really nothing more than an Amazake-based product, which is thinner and less sweet than the traditional variety. The good news is that this product is very similar to milk and can be used in many recipes that call for cow milk. Many supermarkets now carry almond-, rice-, oat-, and potato-based beverages. When these beverages are used, they produce a pleasant tasting, low-fat, nutritionally balanced alternative to dairy.

Remember: to gradually support the detoxification process and lose excess pounds, you should gradually change from animal food such as meat, eggs, and cow milk to vegetable-based protein. You will also reduce bad fats and increase good fats in your diet.

If you use cold-pressed vegetable oils (especially extra-virgin olive and canola), you will be supplying yourself with good essential fatty acids. If you avoid fried foods and broil, bake, or steam your food, you will avoid eating damaging oxygenated fats. And if you steam rather than boil, you will lose fewer nutrients.

Herbal Antioxidants for a Long and Healthy Life

Oxygen is essential to life, but it may also be damaging when it appears in the body in the wrong place and at the wrong time. This damage comes from excess levels of what are known as free radicals. Over the years, studies have shown that even the polyunsaturated fats that have been so aggressively marketed on television can speed up the aging process in the skin, with the result of increased wrinkling about the face. According to Nathan Pritikin, the weight-loss pioneer and the developer of the famous

Pritikin Diet, all fats, including animal and vegetable, have the common effect of causing red blood cells and platelets and other elements in the blood to stick together. One of the results of this clumping is that capillaries and other small blood vessels become clogged and shut down. A good part of the problem with oils can be traced to the highly reactive oxygen that they carry. The heating of oils (and the most natural of oils involves heat in the extraction process), speeds up the oxidation process, resulting in earlier rancidity through the effects of free radicals.

Oxidation is the process of oxygen combining with other compounds in the body. An example is the interaction oxygen has with components of the cell membrane called lipids. This oxidation reaction causes the breakdown of body cells. Oxidation is damaging the DNA, which is the blueprint for all new cells. This damaged DNA then replicates damaged cells over and over again. The oxidation of lipids creates chemicals called peroxides that are damaging to proteins. Lipid peroxidation eventually leads to the formation of free radicals.

Free radicals are impossible to avoid, and not all free radicals are destructive to the system. Some immune systems are made up of them and use them as a protective factor against other foreign invaders. Free radicals may even assist in the breakdown of our foods into nutrients.

Many free radicals come from our external environment, such as chemicals in the air, water, certain medicines, and from dietary patterns that include high-fat foods, fried foods, and foods containing many artificial ingredients. Many of the problems we encounter with free radicals arise when so many of them form in our bodies that they begin to cause damage to the system. This damage may affect essential proteins and cause cells to deteriorate. Among most medical researchers, it is now the general consensus that free radicals are the cause of many modern degenerative diseases, including the aging process.

Scientists have found that specific nutrients called antioxidants can reduce the negative effects of oxidation by stopping or reducing oxidation in those places in the body where it may be harmful.

Oxidation is a good reason for using herbal supplements. There are a number of important herbal and nutritional antioxidants.

Herbal Antioxidants:
1. Turmeric (Circuma longa)
2. Green tea extract (Camellia sinensis)
3. Pine bark and pine needle extract
4. Grapeseed extract

Turmeric: In traditional herbology, this ancient herb has been employed to treat obesity and to stimulate digestion. It is also used to support liver function and to detoxify the liver and to treat jaundice in both Ayurvedic and Chinese herbal medicine.

The active ingredient in turmeric is curcuminoid. This substance increases bile flow into the intestines. This may explain turmeric's cholesterol-lowering properties. Turmeric stimulates both the production of bile and its discharge via the gallbladder and biliary. It is anti-inflammatory for the digestive system. Turmeric can be beneficial for persons with Irritable Bowel Syndrome, colitis, and Crohn's disease. Turmeric decreases inflammation and stagnation of the mucous membranes. Skin conditions such as excema, psoriasis, and acne can benefit from turmeric's detoxifying properties. For digestive problems such as gastritis and acidity, it may help to increase mucous production and to protect the stomach lining. In terms of weight management, turmeric has a warm, bitter taste characteristic of curried foods. It is this taste and warming quality that makes turmeric a thermogenic herb.

Other agents, such as licorice, milk thistle, dandelion root, artichoke, and flavonoids, when used in combination with turmeric, may enhance turmeric's therapeutic effectiveness. Turmeric is not recommended for pregnant women as it can cause uterine stimulation.

These concerns are based upon therapeutic use and may not be relevant to its consumption as a spice.

Green tea: Green tea is the second most consumed beverage in the world (after water). Much green tea goes through a fermentation process to create its familiar taste, color, and aroma. However, it is unfermented green tea that has medicinal properties.

Green tea regulates the appetite and stimulates BAT cells, increasing thermogenesis and burning excess fat and calories. Green tea may also lower fat absorption by the intestines and inhibit excess carbohydrates from being absorbed.

In traditional Chinese medicine, green tea has been recommended for headaches, poor digestion, general toxicity, immune system dysfunction, and a variety of other ailments. In the West, recent studies have found that green tea possesses several disease-fighting qualities such as aiding in the metabolism of fats and fatty tissues; increasing thermogenesis; improving the body's ratio of LDL cholesterol to HDL cholesterol; reducing overall cholesterol levels; reducing blood pressure; and offering a protective role against stroke and heart disease. The polyphenols in green tea have been shown to have cancer-preventive properties—particularly colorectal, digestive, oral, and lung cancer.

Many health problems are caused by the oxidation of free radicals. Free radicals are highly reactive molecules that travel around the body causing chemical reactions, which can damage cells, including those in the heart tissues. It is believed that the abundance of flavonoids and polyphenols found in green tea keep free radicals from oxidizing and are more powerful in reducing free radical formation than other well-known antioxidants, such as vitamins C and E.

Research on the antioxidant capacity of tea showed that not only does the antioxidant activity in dry tea exceed that of twenty-two fruits and vegetables, but the antioxidants start to move rapidly when added to a cup of boiling water. With this evidence, it is now believed that antioxidant levels in the body can be significantly increased by drinking one cup of tea a day. A U.S. study has shown that drinking at least one cup of tea a day can reduce the risk of heart attack by 44 percent *(Journal of Chinese Medicine)*.

The main components of green tea are natural xanthines such as caffeine, theobromine, theophylline, and tannin. The association of tannin with caffeine causes the caffeine to be released slowly into the blood. This is useful since the absorption of caffeine in small doses does not cause the insomnia that large amounts of caffeine might cause. The slimming activity of green tea is probably due to its caffeine content. Caffeine helps in the secretion of adrenaline and keeps it at a high level. It is known that adrenaline is the hormone that frees fatty acids of the adipose tissues. In the early stages of a weight-management program the drinking of green tea will produce a diuretic effect, reducing water retention.

Pine bark extract: The most powerful antioxidants have been shown to be anthocyanidins, also known as OPCs, leucocyanidins, or pycnogenols. Pycnogenol is a natural plant extract made from the bark of the European costal pine, Pinus maritima. Research indicates that it has a protective effect from more than sixty diseases that are linked to the deleterious chemical action of free radicals including cancer, heart disease, and arthritis.

Pycnogenol has been shown to have powerful antioxidant properties like those of vitamin C and E and is fifty times more effective than vitamin E and twenty times more effective than vitamin C as an antioxidant that readily crosses the blood-brain barrier to directly protect brain cells.

Dr. Jacques Masquelier of the University of Bordeaux in France was awarded the U.S. patent for the use of pycnogenol as a free radical scavenger.

Grapeseed extract: Also known as leucocyanidins or pycnogenols, grapeseed extract is a complex of flavonoids (polyphenols) that will help increase intracellular vitamin C levels, decrease capillary permeability and fragility, scavenge oxidants and free radicals, and uniquely bind to collagen structures to allow the collagen structure to remain protected from destructive forces. Grapeseed extract also prevents the release and synthesis of compounds that promote inflammation, such as histamine, serine proteases, prostaglandins, and leukotrienes.

Nutritional Antioxidants

Vitamin A can have a profound effect on the metabolism of the intestinal mucosa, increasing the secretion of mucus and restoring normal barrier function. You can find it abundantly in green, leafy vegetables such as beet tops, collard greens, dandelion greens, mustard greens, Swiss chard, kale, and escarole.

String beans, sweet potatoes, broccoli, green peas, watercress, carrots, tomatoes, red peppers, and yellow squash, as well as apricots, cherries, cantaloupes, avocados, oranges, papayas, bananas, prunes, and yellow peaches are also great sources of vitamin A.

Vitamin C is an important nutritional antioxidant. Studies show that it protects against pollution and cigarette smoke and increases life expectancy.

Vitamin E and selenium often work together as nutritional antioxidants. Vitamin E inhibits inflammation and reduces damage by free radicals.

Lecithin is a phospholipid. Phospholipids are nutrients that play an essential role in tissue cleansing and weight loss. In addition, phospholipids render fats water-soluble. Lecithin is found in wheat, oats, peanuts, and rice, but the most effective source is soybeans.

Soy lecithin, as well as helping the body to get rid of excess fat and accumulated toxins, plays an important role in protecting brain and muscular structure tissues from cell damage due to exposure to radiation and toxic chemicals. Lecithin protects the liver, kidneys, and heart tissue. It also helps to dissolve and regulate blood cholesterol, prevents and diminishes hardening of the arteries, and increases resistance to disease.

Superoxide dismutase is an antioxidant enzyme that protects cells and tissues from free-radical damage.

OPCs and Heart Disease

Many nutritional and herbal antioxidants including both pine needle extract and grapeseed extract are rich in complex agents

L-Glutamine: This powerful growth-hormone inducer eliminates food cravings and also has potent anti-aging properties.

Chromium: Obesity can result from an imbalance of the hormone insulin, whose actions of balancing blood-sugar are enhanced by chromium. Chromium, specifically tri-valent chromium, not only is difficult to get in sufficient amounts through your diet, but also is easily depleted by excess sugar consumption. Levels also decline with age. It can be obtained from nutritional yeast and as a supplement.

Vanadium: Like chromium, vanadium helps in the conversion of carbohydrates to energy instead of fat.

L-Tyrosine: This amino acid improves the burning of fats by increasing your metabolism. It works well with the Bach Remedies since it enhances mood and energy at the same time.

called OPCs. As if to reinforce the necessity of including OPCs in our diets, the respected British Medical Journal, the *Lancet* (March 23, 1996), released in a study that lack of vitamin E was a more consistent predictor of heart disease than high cholesterol levels. The study indicated low levels of vitamin E to be predictive of heart attacks 62 percent of the time, while high cholesterol was predictive only 29 percent of the time. Many researchers believe that this result was due to vitamin E's antioxidant properties.

All these antioxidants are available in health food stores in capsule form and have no side effects.

Combining Herbs: The Whole-Body Tonic

The concept of combining herbs to create a synergistic effect has been used in recent years to support the body in achieving what it needs for optimum performance. Combining the proper herbs for you in the proper manner will open the door to improved physical function and weight loss. For instance, homeopathic flower

> **St. John's Wort (Hypericum perforatum):** This yellow-flowered plant is found in many herbal fen-phen products. Recent studies indicate that it is a mood elevator and may curb overeating associated with depression by increasing production of the brain chemical serotonin. Though it is generally considered safe, there have been some reports of increased eye and skin sensitivity to sunlight, mild fatigue, gastrointestinal distress, dizziness, and itching.

remedies work well with herbs that are calming for the emotions like kava kava or St. John's Wort.

Often, we seek out a one-shot-cure-all wonder substance, whether it is a pill, a chemical, a plant, or a magic elixir. Of course, there is no such wonder drug. However, by carefully selecting the plants and herbs that fit our body and our lifestyle needs, we can produce an effective herbal tonic that can assist our body in losing unnecessary weight.

Herbs can be combined to benefit the immune system, cardiovascular system, digestive system, and energy production. By combining herbs to optimize these important body functions, along with herbs to balance the relationship between your mind, body, and emotions, you can boost your state of health, prevent infectious and non-infectious diseases, cure common ailments, and, of course, lose weight.

Combined herbs can also decrease stress and anxiety, build new muscle tissue, and help keep bowel movements regular. They can help rejuvenate you when you are sick or depressed.

The Healing and Nutrition Power of Herbs and Spices

Nature's gifts, herbs and spices, can heal and detoxify in many different ways. They can be prepared fresh, cooked, sprouted, and juiced.

Herbal weight-loss formulas offer unique benefits in three areas:
1. They can help increase metabolism and burn fat at an accelerated rate.

2. They help cleanse the body by helping the organs cause elimination in a positive manner.

3. They increase emotional stability and the ability to resist the stress that can lead to overeating.

Easily assimilated organic minerals, particularly calcium, silicon, and potassium, found in herbs and spices, help restore mineral and biochemical balance in cells and tissues. And cells and tissues that function properly will be better able to assist you in losing weight.

Mineral imbalances lead to diminished oxygenation, a cause for the disease and premature aging of cells. By supplying needed substances for the body's own healing activity and cell regeneration, herbs will speed you on your way to achieving the weight and look you want.

Nature's own medicines, antibiotics and vegetable hormones, are contained in different herbs, spices, and vegetables. Examples include antibiotic substances present in fresh garlic, onions, tomatoes, and radishes; insulin-like substances in string beans; and hormones contained in both onions and cucumbers needed by the pancreas to produce insulin.

How does one choose the best way of using herbs? Herbal weight-loss products usually come in one of five forms:

1. Herbal teas (loose or tea bags)
2. Air-dried (encapsulated)
3. Freeze-dried (encapsulated)
4. Liquid extracts (alcohol- or glycerin-based)
5. Dried extracts (encapsulated or "solid")

Encapsulated or "solid" dried extracts are the most potent, though liquid extracts are very effective as well.

Herbal Cooking Tips for Body Purification

The way food is prepared can be just as important to health and body purification as the food itself. By using cooking techniques such as the ones below, you can improve the nutritional value of the foods you eat.

Try quick steaming herbs or eating vegetables raw. The natural flavors of herbs, spices, and vegetables are preserved when quick methods of preparation are used.

Be creative in your cooking. Try adding new flavors to foods, such as lemon or lime juice, onions, garlic, green chile, horseradish, cayenne pepper, vinegar, or even a "pinch" of honey.

Unwilling to Cut Meat From Your Diet?

Because of the vast number of toxins found in meat, a vegetarian diet may be the wisest choice, not only for people who want to lose weight, but for most people in general. However, most vegetables do not have all the essential amino acids required to make up a complete protein, which is necessary for a healthy diet. But when two or more are eaten together, their sets of amino acids often will combine to make a complete protein. A meal supplying complete and adequate protein can be had most simply by including grains and beans.

- Use nonstick canola oil sprays for pan frying, stir frying, sautéing, and salad dressings.
- The way food is prepared can be just as important to health and weight control as the food itself. By using cooking techniques such as steaming or broiling, you can improve the nutritional value of the foods you eat.

Dining Out the Healthy Way

1. Ask how foods are prepared, especially about the use of salt, butter, and other saturated fats. Knowing what the chef puts into the dish can help you order wisely.
2. Eat more slowly than you usually do. This can help you recognize when you feel satisfied and can prevent overeating. Stop eating before you feel full; what you don't finish can always be taken home.
3. Order all dishes without butter, cream, heavy sauces, or gravies.

Yerba Maté (Ilex paraguayensis): This herb, commonly called maté, is an evergreen member of the holly family. It grows wild in Argentina, Chile, Peru, and Brazil. Maté was introduced throughout what is now Paraguay and Argentina by the Guarani Indians. It was traditionally used in many of their household cures. In modern Argentina, it is used as a beverage, much as coffee is in the United States.

Yerbe maté contains mateins, a substance belonging to a specialized class of chemical compounds called xanthines. Though only small amounts of these substances occur in maté, they have generated a huge amount of interest due to the fact that though mateins are similar to caffeine, they do not jangle and overstimulate the nervous system and seem to lack most of the negative side effects associated with caffeine. Herbalists claim that maté tea eliminates the sensation of hunger and also cleanses and detoxifies the blood. In addition, it tones the nervous system, restores youthful hair color, retards aging, combats fatigue, stimulates the mind, reduces the effects of debilitating disease, reduces stress, lowers cholesterol, eliminates insomnia, and promotes stamina, endurance, alertness, and strength. It supposedly does all this without side effects and toxicity. It seems to stimulate immunity and is equal or superior as an antioxidant to green tea. It also contains twenty-four vitamins and minerals. In 1964, one group of researchers at the Pasteur Institute and the Paris Scientific Society concluded that maté contains practically all of the vitamins necessary to sustain life.

Benefits of yerba maté to the digestive system:
- Immediate improvement in digestion
- Improved ability of the body to repair damaged and diseased gastrointestinal tissues
- Relief of constipation (even long-term, acute, or chronic)
- Improvement in general bowel muscle function
- Appetite suppressant

Benefits of yerba maté to the nervous system:
- Does not interfere with sleep cycles
- Will help to balance the sleep cycles
- Induces increased rapid eye movement (REM) sleep and even increases the amount of time spent in delta states (deep sleep)

Benefits of yerba maté to the cardiovascular system:
- Growth and repair of the heart is aided by the variety of vitamins and minerals in yerba maté
- Increases the supply of oxygen to the heart during periods of stress
- Assists the body in maintaining aerobic breakdown of carbohydrates (glycolysis) during exercise for extended periods of time. (This assists the body in increasing cardiac efficiency and reducing the buildup of lactic acid during exercise.)
- May reduce blood pressure

4. Skip the creamy salad dressings; instead ask for fresh herbs and oil and vinegar on the side, so that you can control the quantity.
5. Try eat-in natural food restaurants when possible.
6. Share appetizers, entrees, and desserts.
7. Less food on the plate means fewer calories. Ask whether you can get a smaller portion than is usually served.
8. Ask for a dessert of fresh fruit or fruit ice. Your sweet tooth may never know the difference between these and rich, heavy desserts.

Ten Ways to Accelerate Body Purification

1. Eat a variety of fresh, unrefined, and unprocessed foods.
2. If you use sweeteners like honey and maple syrup, do so in moderation.

3. Avoid fat and fatty foods.
4. Avoid caffeine (coffee, iced tea, cola,
   and non-herbal teas).
5. Avoid all alcoholic beverages.
6. Avoid refined white and brown sugar and foods that
   contain them.
7. Eat slowly while sitting down.
8. Choose foods high in complex carbohydrates and high
   quality fiber (such as whole grains and beans).
9. Read labels. Beware of foods that contain artificial colors
   and flavors, preservatives, or high amounts of sodium.
10. Exercise (your body and your imagination!).

Hot Tips

1. Try a cool, full-body ginger herbal sitz bath to increase
   glandular function.
2. Using a drop of eucalyptus oil, massage both earlobes with
   deep, rhythmic pressure in a circular motion before eating.
3. Brush your teeth with a natural cinnamon or peppermint
   toothpaste before eating to decrease appetite.
4. Drink chamomile tea or take some valerian capsules to get
   a good night's sleep to curb overeating.
5. Slow down when you eat. It takes the brain twenty
   minutes to send you the signal that you've eaten enough.
6. Get off of the bus a few blocks early and walk the rest of
   the way.
7. Fix your meals in attractive, Japanese-sized portions, with
   small servings of many different things.

Exercise and Detoxification

Moderate exercise such as thirty minutes of fast walking, bike rid-
ing, jogging, roller-skating, or swimming can greatly enhance the
effects of the detoxifying process. Exercise enhances blood flow to
all the cells of your body, including the fat cells where metabolic
toxins and wastes are stored. Exercise also allows oxygen and

other nutrients to nourish the cells while removing wastes from the blood and lymphatic drainage systems.

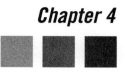

Chapter 4

Losing Weight with Digestive Health

A clean intestinal tract is one of the cornerstones of a successful diet. Unless the intestinal tract is functioning properly, your body won't be functioning properly and you won't reap the benefits of your foods or supplements.

How is your fiber intake? Fiber has been found to have beneficial effects in the realms of nutrition and dieting. Different types of plants have different degrees and kinds of dietary fiber, including cellulose, hemicellulose, pectin, gum, and mucilage.

Insoluble fiber absorbs water as it passes through the digestive system, which increases the speed with which the contents of your intestines pass through your body. It also reduces flare-ups in certain digestive disorders, such as hemorrhoids and constipation.

High-fiber diets may prevent many diseases, including coronary heart disease, colon cancer, diabetes, and diverticulosis. Certain types of fiber also help to decrease blood cholesterol levels.

Pectin and gum can be described as water-soluble fibers that are found in plant cells. They slow down the time it takes for food to pass through your intestines, but they don't do anything to increase fecal bulk. Beans, oat bran, fruits, and vegetables, on the other hand, contain soluble fiber. These types of fiber increase fecal bulk and increase the time it takes for food to pass through the digestive tract.

Wheat bran and whole grains have the largest amounts of insoluble fiber, but beans and vegetables also provide abundant sources.

For optimum health, include a wide variety of high-fiber foods in your diet. You'll find dietary fiber in abundance in fruits, vegetables, nuts, and grains.

Why Fiber Helps You Lose Weight

Fiber itself has no calories, but it gives you a "full" and satisfied feeling because of its ability to absorb water. Take the example of a piece of fruit. Eating the fruit itself will make you feel fuller than an amount of fruit juice with the same number of calories.

And foods with a high-fiber content require a good deal of chewing, so they make a person less likely to consume a large number of calories in a short amount of time.

Insoluble fiber binds water, making stools softer and bulkier to improve elimination. Water-soluble fiber binds bile acids, which seems to suggest that a high-fiber diet will increase the excretion of cholesterol. But some types of fiber have a more intense effect on the body than others. For example, the fiber found in rolled oats seems to be more effective in the lowering of blood cholesterol levels than the fiber found in wheat. Pectin has also been found to lower cholesterol levels in the blood.

Dietery fiber may help decrease the risk of some cancers, especially colon cancer, again because insoluble fiber increases the rate at which wastes are excreted from the body. In other words, the ingestion of fiber reduces the body's exposure to toxins during the digestive process.

Although fiber is crucial to an effective weight-loss diet, it is only one element of a well-balanced diet. Too much fiber may interfere with the amount of calcium, iron, zinc, copper, and magnesium absorbed from your foods.

Where to Get Your Fiber

Plant foods, including fruits, vegetables, nuts, and grains are great sources of dietary fiber. Things such as milk, meat, and eggs contain no fiber. The form in which you ingest a food may or may not affect the amount of its fiber content. Surprisingly, canned and frozen fruits and vegetables have just as much fiber as they do in their natural state. But other types of processing can have an adverse effect on a food's fiber content. Both drying and crushing, for example, destroy fiber's ability to hold water. And any removal of seeds, hulls, or peels will also diminish fiber content.

That is why whole tomatoes have more fiber than peeled tomatoes, which have more fiber than simple tomato juice. And, as we all know, whole-wheat bread contains more fiber than plain white bread.

Fiber supplements come in any number of ways. You can buy simple bran tablets or purified cellulose. In fact, many laxatives sold as stool softeners are fiber supplements.

How much fiber does a person need? There is currently no Recommended Dietary Allowances (RDAs) for fiber, but the average American probably eats about fourteen grams of dietary fiber per day. People with problems such as high cholesterol would probably find some relief if they ate a diet containing up to forty grams of dietary fiber per day. This requires a radical change in eating habits.

Not only must the intake of whole grains, fruits, vegetables, and dried beans increase dramatically, but these changes must take place gradually to prevent problems such as excess gas and diarrhea. (Anyone with a chronic disease should talk to their doctor before making any great changes in their diet.)

Fiber Content on Food Labels

The labels on food reflect public health concerns and now include a daily reference value for specific nutrients, including fiber.

The recommended amount of fiber is twenty-five grams a day based on a two thousand–calorie diet. That would be thirty grams per day based on a twenty-five hundred–calorie diet.

Statements to the effect that something is "made with oat bran" or is "high in oat bran" suggest that the product in question has a substantial amount of oat bran in it. When a statement suggests that an item contains a particular amount of fiber, it can only

Dietary Fiber Content of Foods

Breads, Cereals, Grains		Grams
100% All Bran	⅓ cup	5.1
Corn Flakes	¾ cup	2.3
Cooked Oatmeal	1 cup	1.9
Cooked Brown Rice	⅓ cup	1.6
Cooked White Rice	⅓ cup	0.5
Shredded Wheat	1 biscuit	3.1
White Bread	1 slice	0.7
Whole-Grain Bread	1 slice	2.1

Fruits		
Apples	½ large	2.0
Apricots	2	1.4
Blackberries	½ cup	5.3
Dates	2	1.6
Grapes	10	0.5
Grapefruit	½	0.5
Melons	1	0.5
Nectarines	1	3.3
Oranges	1 small	2.0
Peaches	1	1.6
Pears	1 medium	2.0
Pineapples	½ cup	0.8
Prunes	2	2.4
Raisins	1½ Tbsp.	1.0

Vegetables		
Baked Beans	½ cup	9.3
Green Beans	½ cup	2.1
Beets	½ cup	2.1
Broccoli	½ cup	3.5
Cabbage	½ cup	2.1

Carrots	½ cup	0.4
Cauliflower	½ cup	1.6
Celery	½ cup	1.1
Corn	½ cup	4.7
Lentils, Cooked	½ cup	3.7
Lettuce	½ cup	0.8
Peas	½ cup	1.4
Baked Potato	½ medium	1.9
Sweet Potato	½ medium	2.1
Tomato	1 small	1.5
Winter Squash	½ cup	3.5
Zucchini	½ cup	2.0
Nuts		
Almonds	2 Tbsp.	1.5
Peanuts	2 Tbsp.	0.8

say so if the food really does meet a definition of "high fiber" or a "good source of fiber."

Four High-Protein Body Purifiers

Researchers have found that two types of health bacteria, Lactobacillus acidophilus and Lactobacillus bulgaricus are helpful in both improving digestion and in body detoxification. This bacterium is the same as those used to culture various sour food products, including yogurt. Many individuals use these products as part of their herbal weight-loss program since they are low-fat, high in protein, and improve digestion. Four of the most popular varieties are:

1. Soy or seed yogurt—This is a non-dairy product prepared from soy milk or a combination of seeds and acidophilus. It is generally very sour and is popular primarily with people who want to avoid milk products while receiving the benefits of acidophilus.

2. Buttermilk—Many people believe the myth that buttermilk is high in butter due to its name. The truth is that buttermilk is a wonderfully healing food! It is low in fat, high in protein, and high in calcium. Its rich lactic acid content is also healing to the intestines.

3. Low-fat, skim-milk yogurts—These have less butterfat than whole-milk yogurts (1 percent to 1.5 percent fat). On a weight-management program, the difference between whole-milk and skim milk varieties is about thirty calories per eight-ounce container of unflavored yogurt. When preserves or flavorings are added, the caloric content per cup of plain skim-milk yogurt can increase from about 150 calories to some 250 or more.

4. Kefir—This is a cultured milk drink that virtually all liquid "yogurt drinks" have attempted to copy. Similar to yogurt in taste and nutritional value, kefir in its original form was prepared from mare's milk by nomads in Asia and Russia who drank it as an alcoholic beverage. Commercially available kefir is alcohol-free and is flavored much like yogurt with fruit preserves and sugar. Kefir is thinner than yogurt but still thick enough to spoon out. Most varieties made from low-fat milk have about eighty-five calories in a six-ounce serving of plain and 115 calories if fruited. Kefir has similar virtues as any other dairy product: high-quality protein, calcium, and many of the B vitamins. And, like yogurt, it can be made from low-fat milk.

Note: when buying all food products seek out those that are organically grown, made from non-genetically modified ingredients, and in the case of dairy products, dairy products that are produced from hormone-free milk.

Herbal Teas for Digestive Health

Without healthy digestive function, it is very difficult to begin and maintain a healthy and balanced herbal weight-loss program. Physical discomfort and poor digestive function will result in dietary extremes of excessive food intake or erratic meal schedules.

This section will be especially useful for individuals who suffer from any one of the many physical conditions that might be classified as a digestive disorder. By using a combination of the herbal, nutritional, and homeopathic suggestions that are listed, you may well be able to normalize your digestive function and apply the herbal weight-loss program most effectively.

Digestion

Digestion is the process that food undergoes beginning in the mouth and ending with the elimination of waste materials through the anus. What happens in between these two functions is an amazing array of steps that enables the body to absorb and utilize essential nutrients that nourish the body and eliminate various liquid, solid, and gaseous waste products. In general, we say that digestion begins with chewing. Chewing breaks food into smaller pieces, and saliva breaks down complex carbohydrates and starches. Chewed food passes from the mouth down through the esophagus. Different parts of this long tube perform different functions. Branching off from it are various organs and glands that contribute to digestion, including the pancreas, the liver, and the gallbladder. When any of the many mechanical or chemical processes involved in digestion are stressed or break down, you will experience one or more of the many different symptoms that indicate a digestive disorder including obesity.

Symptoms of Digestive Disorders

Also known as gastrointestinal disorders, digestive problems are often associated with obesity. They begin to make themselves known through symptoms such as cramping, burning, growling, pain, churning, and bloating.

When such symptoms return frequently or become worse, it's time to consult a competent herbalist or other health professional.

You should also consult a professional if you:
- Have difficulty swallowing
- Find blood in your vomit
- Find mucus or pus in your stools
- Experience inexplicable, recurring pain lasting six hours or more accompanied by fever, chills, and shaking
- Experience bowel movement changes, e.g., a sudden change from diarrhea to constipation, or an extreme change in the color of the stool
- Notice a yellowing of the skin and eyes that's not associated with normal beta-carotene supplementation or drinking carrot juice (This is a symptom of jaundice.)
- Notice a dark coloring of the urine that is not associated with a high intake of B vitamins
- Have an unexplained fever of over 101 degrees for two days or more

The most common causes of digestive disorders are:
- Overeating
- Eating too rapidly and not chewing food sufficiently
- Nutritional deficiencies, especially those resulting from ingesting large amounts of refined carbohydrates and other processed foods
- Using coffee, caffeinated tea, alcohol, and tobacco products
- Low levels of hydrochloric acid (possibly the result of a niacin deficiency)
- Very spicy foods

Four Signs That Your Digestion Is in Balance
1. At the end of the day you have a sense of emotional gratification without feeling exhausted
2. You wake up feeling rested after a full night's sleep
3. You have full, easy bowel movements
4. You are able to easily digest your food

How Herbs Can Help Ease Digestive Problems

Herbs can be exceptionally helpful in both preventing and treating digestive disorders. The herbs that are used most often for digestive complaints are licorice, chamomile, peppermint, flaxseed, slippery elm, and aloe vera. The following herbs are used for more specific problems:

Heartburn: ginger, caraway seed, fennel, sage, fresh celery stalks, chamomile, dandelion, and yarrow

Abdominal pains and colic in children: catnip, fennel, peppermint, lobelia, anise, and ginger

Also for colic, try a daily mixture of three cups of chamomile and fennel, mixed half and half.

Colitis: slippery elm gruel

Dyspepsia: gentian, chamomile flowers, angelica root, and lemon balm

Nausea: oat straw, slippery elm bark, and ginger

Also for nausea, try two cups a day of a mixture of raspberry leaf, ginger root, peppermint leaf, and lemon balm.

Ulcers: slippery elm gruel, whole licorice root

Nutrition for Digestive Health

Many people who have struggled with eating disorders and have a history of yo-yo dieting may also experience the symptoms of various digestive disorders. Various herbal and natural healing approaches can be very helpful in such conditions. Here are some things to think about:

Avoid spicy herbs and foods: When you are suffering from a digestive disorder, avoid spicy foods and herbs, coffee, green and black teas, and alcohol. In acute conditions, avoid high-fiber foods.

Try cultured foods: Cultured foods prevent intestinal putrefaction, and are very effective healers for those suffering from virtually any digestive problems. Cultured foods include sauerkraut, kefir, sourdough bread, yogurt, and buttermilk.

> **Guggulipid:** Guggul is a gummy resin that oozes from a tree (Commiphora mukul) that grows in India. Used for other disorders, guggulipid contains plant compounds called guggulsterones that have been proven to regulate the metabolism. Guggulipid also stimulates the BAT cells, thereby increasing thermogenesis and burning stored fat.
>
> One medically accepted study conducted in India in 1994 showed that daily doses of one hundred milligrams of guggulipid effectively reduced LDL ("bad") cholesterol and triglycerides.
>
> Pregnant women and people with thyroid disorders, as well as those on medications such as calcium channel blockers, should not take guggulipid, nor should women with menstrual problems. Possible side effects include excessive menstrual bleeding and digestive disorders, such as nausea, vomiting, and diarrhea.

Add fiber: Many gastrointestinal disorders can be traced to the patient's diet, specifically to diets high in refined foods and low in essential fiber. A vegetarian low-fiber diet is best when the condition is inflamed, but after this acute stage, a high-fiber diet is best. Raw bran, whole grains, and beans are good sources of dietary fiber, but they should be taken in moderation and with plenty of fluids. To avoid complications, be sure to limit your use of bran to two to five tablespoons daily.

Drink distilled or highly purified spring water: If you have digestive problems, drink distilled water. Any of the many different chemicals in tap water might aggravate or possibly cause a digestive problem.

Eat plenty of vegetable salads: At the end of a meal, especially after eating proteins, be sure to eat salads. The salad will enable the protein-digesting acids and enzymes to function without interference from carbohydrates, which are digested by other enzymes.

Specialized food combining: For some individuals, mixing many different types of food at the same meal can aggravate their symptoms. If this applies to you, avoid mixing fruits, vegetables,

Wall Germander (Teucrium chamaedrys L., Labiatae):
This flowering plant was recognized by ancient herbalists as a bitter tonic for its stimulating influence on the digestive functions. Europeans have also found the herb to be of value as part of various weight-reducing regimens, helping to stimulate the reduction of fatty deposits and cellulite. It is a complement in weight-loss programs thanks to its tannin content, which allows a decrease in fatty deposits.

grains, and beans at the same meal. Limit the combination of many different foods or carbohydrates and proteins at the same meal.

Nutritional and Herbal Solutions to Digestive Disorders
Abdominal Gas
To reduce abdominal gas, follow these suggestions:
1. Eliminate raw fruits and vegetables for a while, and instead, drink fresh vegetable juices and eat lower-fiber foods such as peeled fruits, bananas, and avocados.
2. Avoid foods that are known to cause gas, like bananas, milk, cucumbers, beans, peas, and vegetables in the cabbage family (broccoli, cauliflower, and Brussels sprouts).
3. Use activated charcoal capsules. When used in moderation, charcoal is very effective in eliminating gas, but excessive use can deplete essential minerals from your system.

Colitis
With this condition, a high-fiber diet is not necessarily recommended, especially if the source of fiber is whole grain. In cases of colitis, the roughage is poorly digested and can cause fermentation in the bowels, resulting in gas and bowel irritation.

Eat small meals several times a day rather than a few large meals. Eat yogurt and millet, and experiment by including bananas in your diet on a regular basis. You may want to try a juice fast for a week or so, especially in the case of mucous colitis.

Diarrhea

If you suffer from diarrhea, raw carrots can be very helpful. Cinnamon, ginger, slippery elm bark powder, thyme tea, and extracts of yarrow, plantain, and red raspberry leaf added to water may be of help.

Diverticulosis

To avoid diverticular disease, avoid constipation. Eat high-fiber foods like millet, brown rice, buckwheat, oats, and foods rich in lactic acid such as sauerkraut, kefir, etc.

Heartburn

To fight off the effects of heartburn, eat unprocessed raw miller's bran. Extracts of wood betony, willow, and angelica added to water may be of help. Also, be sure to avoid alcohol, chocolate, coffee (both decaffeinated and regular coffee), tobacco products, citrus fruits, fried foods, spicy foods and herbs, and tomatoes and foods containing tomatoes. (The nicotine in tobacco products aggravates heartburn by forcing sphincter pressure to drop, allowing a bringing up of stomach acid. Avoid smoking.)

Hiatal Hernia

Avoid all products containing caffeine. Avoid alcohol, spicy foods, and high-fat foods.

Lactose Intolerance

Avoid milk and milk products except those foods with reduced lactose levels, such as buttermilk, yogurt, cottage cheese, and kefir. In fact, you should even limit the amount of lactose-reduced foods that you consume. Whenever you do consume lactose-rich foods, take tablets that will counteract their effects.

Ulcers

If you have ulcers, there are a number of general recommendations you should heed whenever the condition is active. Avoid high-fiber foods, including raw fruits and vegetables, whole grains, breads, seeds, and cereals. In addition, avoid coffee, alcohol, tobacco products, and milk. Although milk may initially coat the stomach lining, it will also decrease stomach acid and aggravate the situation.

> **Ginger (Zingiber officinale):** A perennial, ginger grows in Asia, Mexico, Jamaica, and other countries. Its underground stem, the rhizome, has been widely used in traditional Chinese medicine for the treatment of inflammatory joint diseases such as arthritis and for various digestive conditions such as vomiting, diarrhea, coughing, and abdominal bloating. Ginger increases blood circulation, aids in the metabolism of dietary nutrients, and plays an important role in Ayurvedic treatments as well. As a digestive tract tonic, ginger stimulates digestion and tones the intestinal muscles. It has a carminative effect; it aids in the break up and expulsion of intestinal gas. Ginger has also been shown to reduce nausea and prevent motion sickness.
>
> Ginger may also act as an antioxidant. Antioxidants slow the rate at which free radicals and other fats combine with oxygen and become rancid. Decocted as a tea, it helps to cleanse the digestive and circulatory systems. It is currently popular as a treatment in the early stages of a cold or the flu. Ginger oil is also very popular as a healing tool in aromatherapy.

Do not fast during an active or acute phase of ulcers.

These foods should be tolerable: avocados, yams, bananas, white potatoes, and squash. Also, you might try this: blend a handful of blanched almonds with a little barley malt syrup and distilled water. Pour the blend through a strainer. Drink the remaining liquid.

For duodenal ulcers, olive oil—one tablespoon three times a day for as long as one year—can be helpful.

Extracts of wood betony, willow, and angelica added to water may be of help.

Certain types of fiber both prevent the formation of ulcers and, at the same time, prevent relapses. The foods that best provide this type of fiber are millet, raw miller's bran, and beans.

Remember that these foods should not be eaten during the active phase of duodenal ulcers.

If you have ulcerative colitis, food allergies may be contributing to your condition. Avoid milk products, wheat, corn, oats, barley, and rye.

An herbal combination containing Pau d'Arco, clove powder extract, Inula racemosa, deglycyrrihizinated licorice extract, and Capsicum has been found to contain antibacterial properties ideal for inhibiting the activity of Helicobacter pylori bacteria, also referred to as H. pylori. This is the bacteria that has been found to cause ulcers. Unlike most bacteria inhibitors, these herbs do not inhibit the effects of good intestinal bacteria.

Nutritional Supplements for Digestive Disorders

Colitis: vitamins A and C, folate, zinc, and pantothenic acid

These healing nutrients are, interestingly, the same nutrients that are found to be deficient in colitis sufferers.

Flatulence: pantothenic acid

Heartburn: combination of sodium alginate and calcium/magnesium tablets

Peptic Ulcers: follow the nutritional recommendations in the section on Hypoglycemia.

Many people who suffer from peptic ulcers also have hypoglycemia.

Ulcers: vitamins A and E taken together, supplement with zinc

Juice Therapy for Digestive Problems

For all gastrointestinal disorders, you may take Juice Therapy Formulas No. 1 and No. 4 (see chapter 8). In addition, you may drink fresh papaya, wheat grass, pineapple, or lemon juice. If you wish, try mixing whey with your juices, or buy Biota brand juices, which already contain whey.

Amoebic Dysentery: garlic juice

Colitis: papaya juice and raw cabbage juice

Also, follow the juice program for ulcers, listed next. Avoid citrus juices.

Ulcers: combine twelve ounces of carrot juice with four ounces of cabbage juice and drink the mixture once a day for one week. After one week, slowly increase the amount of cabbage juice in the mixture from four to twelve ounces. Also, mix raw potato and cabbage juice and drink the combination immediately after extraction. Otherwise, the mixture loses the healing value.

Constipation and Ulcers: five times a day, drink three ounces of celery juice mixed with three ounces of cabbage juice. Also, each day drink one pint of spinach juice, the most powerful juice for relieving constipation.

Sluggish and Prolapsed Colon: drink sorrel juice, which is available at Jamaican food stores.

Accupressure, Herbal Oils, and Massage

Try accupressure and massage for digestive disorders.

For general disorders, try kneading the abdomen. Also, massage along the dorsal and lumbar spine with oil of lavender or jasmine.

To treat gastric ulcers, apply deep rhythmic pressure to both wrists.

Understand and Control Emotional Factors to Help Digestive Disorders

Depression or fear can slow down your digestive activity. On the other hand, anger can increase the secretion of acid into the stomach and this excess acid can break down the stomach wall and cause ulcers. Learn and use the techniques discussed in this book to control your emotions.

Homeopathic Remedies for Digestive Disorders

Homeopathy is a system of medicine that is based on what is known as The Law of Similars. The truth of this law has been verified experimentally and clinically for the last two hundred years. Samuel Hahnemann, the founder of modern homeopathy, described this principle by using a Latin phrase *Similia Similibus Curentur*, which translates: "Let likes cure likes." Hahnemann developed the principle into a system of medicine he called homeopathy. Many homeopathic remedies, especially for digestive disorders, are prepared from herbs.

Problem	Homeopathic Remedy
General Digestive Problems	arsenicum
Indigestion	bryonia
Abdominal Gas	chamomilia
Vomiting Blood	arsenicum
Vomiting Caused by Overeating	antimonium crudum

Tissue Salt Remedies

Tissue salts, also known as cell salts, are vibrationally based homeopathically prepared remedies. They were developed by Wilhelm Heinrich Schuessler, a German physician in the nineteenth century. According to Schuessler, these remedies, of which there are twelve, eliminate deficiencies of the vital inorganic elements that are essential to life. They are available in many health food stores and pharmacies that sell nutritional and homeopathic products.

Try the following tissue salts for digestive disorders:

Colic: magnesium phosphate 6X with warm water every ten minutes until pain subsides

Improving Poor Digestion: calcium phosphate 6X and potassium phosphate 6X

After Eating Rich, Fatty Foods: alternate taking potassium chloride and phosphate of iron

Heartburn and Yellow-Coated Tongue: sodium phosphate.

If this doesn't work, take these together: magnesium phosphate, sodium phosphate, sodium sulphate, and silicic oxide.

Flatulence and Colic: magnesium phosphate with hot fennel or ginger tea.

If this does not work, take these together: calcium phosphate, magnesium phosphate, sodium phosphate, and sodium sulfate.

Nausea and Vomiting: sodium sulfate 6X or phosphate of iron

The Pancreas and the Glycemic Index

One of the most hidden of the digestive disorders concerns the relationship between the pancreas and a scale of how foods are metabolized. This scale is commonly known as the glycemic index. It is difficult to develop a successful weight-loss program without paying attention to the pancreas and glycemic index. The pancreas is a gland with multiple functions, among them being the important task of producing insulin in amounts geared to the quantity of sugar entering the body and how much of this sugar should be allowed into the blood stream. The glycemic index is a means for measuring the effect an individual food has on these blood sugar (glucose) levels. The index has been utilized for years by diabetics and hypoglycemics as a way to predict how their bodies will respond to certain foods. With this approach, it is easier to control their diets and develop healthy meal plans.

In recent years, a number of dietary programs have begun to see the value of using the glycemic index as an effective tool for taking weight off and keeping it off. Like any other valid information, the glycemic index can be used to extremes and cause other problems, but when used responsibly, it is a valuable tool for making effective food choices and reducing food cravings.

The organization of the index revolves around the ranking of glucose at an arbitrary figure of 100. Foods are evaluated by how fast they turn into blood sugar in comparison to sucrose. Foods with a glycemic index above 100 turn into blood sugar even faster than sucrose. The higher the ranking of the food the more glycemic it is. A food whose glycemic ranking is over 60 is considered high on the glycemic index. The higher a food ranks on the glycemic index, the greater its influence on glucose levels.

The importance of the glycemic index in developing an effective weight-management program is tied to the complex and at times controversial issue of insulin resistance. It is generally accepted among nutrition and weight-loss experts that insulin resistance is an underlying cause of obesity, unhealthy blood fat profiles, and adult-onset diabetes. Eating excessive amounts of high-ranking glycemic foods places unnecessary stress on the pancreas. This stress can create insulin resistance in the long run.

The controversial response of some nutrition experts to the excessive attention to the glycemic index has to do with the promotion of various diet and weight-loss regimes that recommend high protein intake, and not only the low-fat approach to dieting but extremely low carbohydrate intake as well. Interestingly, how you plan your meals may influence the glycemic index. The glycemic index is generally lower for foods that are minimally processed and are ingested along with fat and protein.

Exercise also has an impact on how the glycemic index of a food will affect an individual. Research has found that consumption of lower glycemic index foods thirty to sixty minutes prior to an aerobic exercise tends to reduce the hypoglycemia that occurs at the start of exercise, supresses the insulin response to carbohydrate ingestion (it is suppressed during exercise), increases the concentration of fatty acids in the blood, increases fat oxidation, and reduces reliance on carbohydrate fuel.

Factors that influence the glycemic index of a food include the biochemical structure of the carbohydrate, the absorption process, the size of the food particle, the degree of thermal processing, the contents and timing of the previous meal, and the co-ingestion of fat, fiber, or protein, ripeness of the food, time of day eaten, cooking time, and amount of heat used in cooking, blood insulin levels, and an individual's recent physical activity.

Mechanical processing, or processing of food that involves heat or that breaks the food into smaller particles or makes it more susceptible to the actions of the digestive enzymes, increases the glycemic index of the food. For example, eating foods prepared from wheat flour will increase the glycemic index relative to ingesting wheat kernels. Since ingestion of protein slows the amount of time it takes for the stomach to empty, absorption of carbohydrates and elevations in blood glucose generally occur more slowly if the carbohydrates are consumed along with fats and proteins.

Blood glucose may affect how great a person's appetite may be and even allow them to control it better since diets composed of low glycemic index foods may increase the dieter's sense of fullness. Since blood glucose appears to be so critical to the eating patterns and food choices of those on weight-management programs, the charts I have included may help you to make more effective food choices. Though the research is in the beginning stages, it seems that a low-glycemic index diet, combined with the use of thermogenic herbs, is a good choice for an effective and healthy herbal weight-loss program.

Glycemic Index for Common Foods

Low GI means a smaller rise in blood sugar and less stress on the pancreas. These glycemic index numbers are an approximation based on a combination of the numbers listed from a many different research labs and from various studies. Thus numbers on various glycemic index lists will be similar but not necessarily exactly the same.

These numbers are based on glucose, which is the fastest absorbed carbohydrate available except for maltose. Glucose is given a value of 100 and all other carbohydrates are given a number relative to glucose.

The Glycemic Index
Green Leafy Vegetables

With rare exception, green leafy vegetables are very low on the glycemic index and can be used as you wish, though even these should be eaten with portion control.

Fruits		Legumes	
Apple	36	Baby Lima Beans	32
Banana (unripe)	30	Baked Beans	48
Cantaloupe	65	Black Beans	30
Cherries	22	Butter Beans	31
Grapes	52	Chick Peas	33
Kiwi	52	Kidney Beans	27
Mango	55	Lentils	29
Orange	43	Navy Beans	38
Papaya	58	Pinto Beans	42
Peach	42	Soy Beans	18
Pear	36	Split Peas	82
Pineapple	66		
Plum	24	**Starchy Vegetables**	
Raisins	64	Carrots	71
Watermelon	72	Green Peas	48
		Potatoes, Baked	83
		Potatoes, Mashed	73
		Sweet Potatoes	54

Dairy

Dairy can be a little complex concerning the glycemic index. Full-fat milk, for example, has a rating of 27, while skim milk has a rating of 32. This happens because the percentage of lactose (milk sugar) in skim milk increases when the fat is removed. We want less saturated fat, but we also want a lower GI rating. My suggestion is to use soy milk (a 31 GI rating) or rice beverages. Even if some are a little on the higher side of the GI rating, they are saturated fat free.

Breads and Grains

(Though I do not recommend using them, I have included some popular commercially refined grain-based breakfast cereals.)

All Bran	42	Millet	75
Bagel	72	Muesli	60
Barley	25	Oatmeal	61
Bran Muffin	60	Popcorn	55
Bread, Whole Wheat	69	Puffed Wheat	25
Buckwheat	54	Rice Bran	19
Bulgur	47	Rice Cakes	82
Cheerios	74	Rice Krispies	82
Corn Flakes	77	Rice, Brown	55
Cornmeal	68	Rice, Instant	91
Couscous	65	Rice, White	56
Doughnut	76	Rolled Oats (oatmeal)	49
Gnocchi	68	Rye	63
Grape Nut Flakes	80	Shredded Wheat	69
Grape Nuts	67	Spaghetti, White	41
Hominy	40	Waffle	76
Life Cereal	66	Wheat Bread, White	70
Macaroni and Cheese	64	Wheat Kernels	41
Macaroni	46	Whole Wheat	37

Miscellaneous Snacks

Most snack foods, including candy, potato chips, corn chips, and other highly processed and refined foods, are undesirable as part of any diet. So, I have chosen not to include them on this glycemic index list.

Chocolate	49	Peanuts	14

Sugars

Fructose	23	Honey	58
Lactose	46	Sucrose	65

Foods "high" on the index, some of which are not listed here, include: ice cream, croissants, potatoes, bread, raisins and other dried fruit, bananas, carrots, and watermelon. Foods that rank as moderate on the glycemic index (between 45 and 60) include most types of pasta, bulgur, baked beans, yams, green peas, sweet potatoes, orange juice, blueberries, and rice. Low glycemic index foods, the ones you will want to use (ranking under 45), include beans, cruciferous vegetables, and high-fiber, low-sugar cereals as well as low-fat, unsweetened, plain yogurt, grapefruit, apples, and tomatoes, to name a few.

I have found the most effective approach to integrating the glycemic rating system in an herbal-based, weight-management system includes:

1. Paying attention to portion control.
2. Using whole-grain breads made with whole seeds.
3. Using whole-grain pasta and even pasta made from unbleached white flour or brown rice in place of potatoes.
4. Choosing whole-grain breakfast cereals based on wheat bran, barley, and oats.
5. Using lemon juice and vinegar dressings.
6. Mixing 30 percent of total calories from vegetarian proteins with 40 to 50 percent from carbohydrates ranked low to moderate on the glycemic index. Fat calories should be in the 20 to 25 percent range and should be derived from monounsaturates such as olive oil.
7. Using herbal formulas and nutrients that strengthen pancreatic function.

Chapter 5

Reducing Food Cravings with Aromatherapy

Aromatherapy is one of the most powerful tools available for reducing food cravings and creating a sense of emotional and sensory satisfaction that most of us would normally get by eating.

Of the five senses, the sense of smell and taste are unique. They are chemically based senses, in that they sense chemicals, and all smells are, of course, chemicals. It is with these two senses that we can investigate our surrounding environment for chemical information. Many researchers in the field of aromatherapy believe that smell can influence memory, mood, food choices, mate choice, the immune system, and the production of hormones.

There are two mechanisms through which smell affects our emotions, moods, and physiology: memory and contextual association, and the intrinsic pharmacological properties of the odor molecule itself.

Throughout this chapter you will learn to understand weight loss, aromatherapy, and your emotions. I have placed brief outlines of some of the most common aromatherapy oils and the herbs that have been extracted. Some have more detailed descriptions available, especially when these herbs are used in cooking and food preparation.

Weight Loss, Your Emotions, and Aromatherapy

As you develop and apply new eating patterns, you may find yourself occasionally feeling deprived. After all, you are giving up

Mugwort Oil (Armoise, Artemisa vulgaris): A great assistant to promoting vivid dreams, it is also used to regulate and balance female cycles and promote one's psychic powers.

Allspice Oil (Pimenta dioica, Pimenta officinalis): Allspice is the fruit of an evergreen tree native to Jamaica and parts of Central and South America. In flavor it tastes like a combination of cinnamon, cloves, juniper berries, and other spices, hence its name. The key chemical constituent, eugenol, is an oil that is the primary source of the herb's flavor. Eugenol is also an antiseptic and a fungicide. Historically, herbalists used allspice as a poultice for the relief of arthritis pain. The allspice oil is valuable as part of a weight-management program for its ability to reduce indigestion and flatulence.

Dried, whole allspice berries are used in pickling liquids and in spicing drinks. Ground allspice works well in cakes, pies, and other desserts.

old habits for new, healthy lifestyle patterns. Old habits and long-established patterns are simply hard to break. This can be very frustrating. Everyone experiences frustration. How you deal with it will determine its impact on you.

Radical changes in eating and exercise habits are very difficult and nearly impossible to achieve in less than five or six months. Frustration can be used broadly as a general term to describe such things as irritation, anxiety, stress, and impatience. Babies cry out of frustration, and because they cannot communicate the problem; they are usually given a bottle or nipple to comfort them.

As adults, we have been conditioned to believe that temper tantrums are unacceptable, so reverting back to an early life pattern, we may reach for food in an attempt to comfort ourselves. Even when we do eat to relieve frustration and depression, we usually go for the foods we ate as a child, such as

Basil Oil (Ocimum basilicum): An uplifting oil, basil is an adrenal that clears the mind, improves memory, helps in concentration, and focuses the senses. It is soothing for those who are fearful, particularly of intimacy. It works nicely with the Bach Remedies. (Remember: oils are inhaled, Bach Remedies are taken orally.) Basil has been used historically to combat anxiety, depression, and insomnia. It is also useful in the treatment of addictions, fatigue, colds, migraines, and headaches. Do not use it in large doses since it can make you feel a little drunk or woozy. Commonly referred to as "sweet basil" or "garden basil," this classic kitchen spice adds a refreshingly warm flavor to foods. Do not use the aromatic oil when pregnant.

Lemon Oil (Citrus limonum): Extracted from lemon peels, this cool, refreshing oil tones the circulatory system. Emotionally, it brings clarity to the mind and reduces depression. The main constituents of lemon oil are limonene, terpinene, pinene, myrcene, citral, linalol, geraniol, and citronellal. Through these constituents, lemon oil has a beneficial effect on the immune system and increases detoxification through the skin by stimulating the lymphatics and by reducing water retention.

Lemon oil blends well with orange flower, violet, bergamot, citronella, neroli, and galbanum. A combination of these oils are popular in beauty care due to their cleansing, refreshing, astringent, antiseptic, and cooling qualities.

Warning: lemon oil may cause photosensitivity. Do not use before exposure to the sun.

sweets, because our brains associate the food with relieving the problem.

Aromatherapy, the name used to describe the various therapeutic applications of essential oils, may help you reduce this sense of frustration and deprivation. The French doctor and scientist Rene-Maurice Gattefosse is credited with coining the

Lavender Oil (Lavendula angustifolia): Lavender is one of the most versatile oils and is extremely popular in weight-management programs. Extracted from the flowering tops of the plant, this floral and mildly camphorous oil, which is produced primarily in France, is calming, soothing, and great for insomnia, nervous anxiety, fear, melancholy, and stress. Its main constituents are linalol, linalyl acetate, lavandulol, lavandulyl acetate, terpineol, limonene, and caryophyllene. It is antifungal and antibacterial, and great for treating burns, cuts, bruises, and other skin irritations. This highly versatile oil is a stimulant for the immune system. Its light, clear, flowery aroma aids sleep, soothes tired muscles, and encourages tranquility and calm.

Lavender blends well with so many oils and has so many uses that they are too numerous to list. It blends especially well with clove, rose, jasmine, rosemary, eucalyptus, patchouli, and bergamot.

Warning: do not use during pregnancy.

Mandarin Orange Oil (Citrus reticulata): This fruit was once a traditional gift offered to the Chinese Mandarins, hence its name. The oil is obtained by expression from the peels of Indian fruits, and its main constituents are geraniol, linomene, citronellal, and citral.

Used much like lavender oil, this tangy and fruity oil has a gently cheering effect and creates youthful feelings and thoughts. Mandarin oil has a calming effect upon the digestive system. It is a gentle oil, valuable for massage and for balancing the digestive system. A soothing agent, astringent, and skin conditioner, mandarin oil blends well with geranium, grapefruit, bergamot, chamomile, clary sage, basil, olibanum, neroli, orange, rose, lavender, and lemon lime.

Do not use mandarin on the skin in direct sunlight.

name aromatherapy. Though he is considered the twentieth-century father of modern aromatherapy, there is evidence from the great civilizations of the past indicating that the use of herbs

Lemongrass Oil (Cymbopogon citratus): Frequently found in Thai, Vietnamese, and Chinese cooking, most lemongrass oil is extracted by steam distillation from plants that grow in Guatemala. A refreshing, cleansing, and stimulating tonic to the body, it is sometimes added to shampoos. Its refreshing, powerful, sweet lemony aroma may function as an appetite suppressant. Its main constituents are citral, linalol, geraniol, and dipentene. Together they create an aroma that makes an effective muscle relaxant as well as a good deodorizing room fragrance.

The lemongrass herb is also a key ingredient in Indonesian curries. In addition, lemongrass makes a relaxing tea, which may be used as a digestive stimulant. Lemongrass blends well with jasmine, lavender, and geranium.

Bergamot Oil (Bergamot citrus bergamia): The sweet, delicate aroma of this oil is uplifting, refreshing, and useful for those who have anxiety, high stress, and experience depression. This oil is valuable for those whose overeating patterns are a result of grief, sadness, or a great emotional loss. Bergamot increases mental alertness and may correct emotional imbalances. Some researchers believe it may help people break the smoking habit.

Do not place directly on the skin prior to prolonged exposure to the sun.

and aromatics in ancient times was common, and that a large body of knowledge existed concerning the properties of these plants.

Dr. Gattefosse's main achievement was discovering the powerfully antiseptic nature of many essential oils. He also discovered that essential oils are more powerful in their natural state when their active chemicals are used in isolation. Gattefosse recorded the results of his findings in his book *Aromatherpie*, published in 1937.

The Ancient Egyptians applied their knowledge of aromatic plants to almost all aspects of life. They used them for healing, as

Myrrh Oil (Commiphora myrrha resin): This mysterious, smoky oil is rich in heerabolene, limone, dipentene, pinene, and eugeno. It is derived from a tree resin and has a centering quality that assists in emotional centering, visualization, and meditation. It is one of the oldest-known aromatic materials, especially in incense. It is often used in combination with frankincense and also blends well with lavender, patchouli, sandalwood, olibanum, galbanum, and clove.

Marjoram Oil (Origanum majorana): Popular with the ancient Greeks, this spicy, comforting oil is generally derived through steam distillation of the flowering tops of Spanish plants. Oil of marjoram helps create a warm sensation, has a regulating, calming, sedative effect, and is effective for relieving insomnia, stress, and nervous tension. It can be mixed in sweet almond oil to create massage oil for tired muscles, and has been used by many aromatherapists for massaging the abdomen during menstruation. It is pleasant when added to a hot bath, especially blended with any combination of equal amounts of chamomile, cypress, cedarwood, lavender, or mandarin. Many people overeat to soften the grief and loneliness that comes with the loss of a loved one. Marjoram oil is an excellent alternative. Sweet marjoram, as marjoram is sometimes also called, is an excellent seasoning to keep on hand for cooking a variety of dishes.

Warning: do not use this oil excessively during pregnancy.

ingredients in cosmetics, and in burial rituals such as mummification. A papyrus dating back to 1550 B.C., unearthed in 1875, details the recipes for treating a variety of ailments, which are similar to the remedies we would use today.

The Chinese also used aromatics for religious practices as well as for health, and applied them during massage as an additional means of maintaining a healthy body. The Chinese knowledge of herbs in 2500 B.C. is documented in *The Yellow Emperor's Classic of*

Canadian Balsam Oil: Useful as a diuretic, balsam is an antiseptic, relieves coughing, and helps to expel mucus. Used for asthma, bronchitis, catarrh, and sore throat, it also assists in the healing of burns, wounds, and scars. It is useful in promoting weight loss by reducing nervous tension and softening any sense of depression that might arise.

Internal Medicine, written by the Emperor Kiwang-Ti. More than four thousand years later, after twenty-six years of study, Li Shih-Chen published the *Pen Tsao*, an enormous and valuable volume in which he recorded the use of two thousand herbs and twenty essential oils. His book documents the greatest range of herbs studied in any tradition.

In India, the traditional Ayurvedic medical practice was developed from two thousand-year-old texts, which list seven hundred useful aromatics, all valued for their spiritual and health-giving properties. There, as in China, the principal aspect of this form of medicine was the aromatic massage.

Aromatic substances were one of the earliest traded goods, rare and highly prized. Phoenician merchants spread the trade of aromatics into the Arabian Peninsula and across the Mediterranean to Greece and Rome. The Greek physician Marestheus first recorded the stimulating and sedative qualities of different aromatic flowers. In the first century A.D., Dioscorides compiled the *Herbstius*, a five-volume study of the sources and uses of plants and aromatics. This became the standard medical treatise for the following thousand years.

Distilling

Revolutionary developments in science that began during the Renaissance led to the analysis and study of an increasing number of essential oils and other aromatic substances. The famous perfume industry in Grasse, France, developed, and by the end of the seventeenth century, the distinction between apothecaries, who

> **Juniper (Juniperus communis.):** Juniper oil is generally steam distilled from flowers grown in the former Yugoslavia. Psychologically good for low energy, anxiety, and weakness, it is an oil that is historically used with men. Among the most popular of oils among practitioners of the esoteric arts, juniper's woodsy scent is believed to restore psychic purity. Its main constituents include borneol, camphene, pinene, termenic alcohol, myrcene, and thugene, and together they seem to have an influence on physical purification and detoxification. Juniper berry oil helps reduce the effect of emotional overload and is beneficial physically for building immunity and reducing the negative affects of arthritis, rheumatism, sore muscles, acne, ulcers, and varicose veins. Juniper oil blends well with clary sage, cypress, lavandin, and elemi.
>
> Warning: do not use during pregnancy.

dealt with herbs for medicinal purposes, and the perfume manufacturers was quite pronounced.

The advent of mechanized printing meant that the publication of information on popular herbs became possible, making herbal texts available to a wider public.

Such changes provided a background against which modern aromatherapy could develop. In seventeenth-century England, Nicholas Culpeper, John Parkinson, and John Gerarde, among others, led the way in what was the golden age of English herbalism. At the same time, the natural philosophy that had been such an important part of the alchemists' work was left behind to be developed in isolation by artists and thinkers. This development marked the beginning of the separation of body and spirit that is so evident in medical practice today.

During this time, as scientific knowledge about essential oils grew, their use in medicine became less important, and the concept of holism was lost, albeit temporarily. In the mid-seventeenth century, the separation between traditional herbalists and physicians who favored chemical drug therapy began. However, at the

Chamomile Oil (Anthemis nobilis): This apple-scented oil is soothing, calming, and reduces the sense of fatigue that some dieters experience in their muscles both from the shift in body weight and from new exercises that may be part of this program. Chamomile is also calming and soothing to sensitive skin, insomnia, headaches, irritability, and migraines. It also encourages emotional and mental serenity. A particularly popular oil is blue chamomile. This oil contains azulene, which gives it a deep blue color. Azulene promotes new skin cell regeneration and is thus used in skincare preparations.

Chamomile is a popular herbal tea that is a great after-meal beverage. It soothes the digestion and calms the nerves when you are tense.

same time, philosophers exploring alchemy further refined the art of distillation, allowing more and more aromatic essences to be created for a wide range of uses.

The Modern Art and Practice

Many of those who came after Dr. Gattefosse helped to rediscover the link between the mind, spirit, and healthy body. The Frenchman Jean Valnet, also a doctor and scientist, used essential oils to treat wounds during World War II, as well as to treat specific illnesses. Today in France, there are many medical doctors prescribing essential oils for internal use to heal ailments.

Aromatherapy has also been found useful in helping to heal various digestive disorders. Although we usually think of digestion as starting with the mouth, to be even more specific, the process begins the moment that we smell the foods we are about to eat. The aroma stimulates our digestive juices, and the better foods smell, the more enjoyable they will taste and the more digestible they will be.

Herbs and spices not only help to make foods taste better, they also make them smell better.

Myrtus communis (Family, Myrtaceae): Extracted from the flowering tops of this plant through steam distillation, this camphoraceous oil is helpful in meditation, for enlivening a mood of hopelessness, and for freeing clogged sinuses and breathing passages. Myrtus oil was traditionally used by herbalists on the skin as a soothing agent, astringent, skin conditioner, and muscle relaxant.

Myrtus oil blends well with lemongrass, rosemary, bergamot, cardamon, spearmint, thyme, tea tree, lavender, and lemon.

Rosewood (Aniba rosaedora): This pleasant, relaxing, flowery aroma is useful for reducing a sense of depression and establishing emotional clearing and centering. For keeping to your eating program and handling mood swings there are few more useful oils than this woody, floral scent. Balancing, grounding, comforting, and stabilizing are just a few of the words that describe its influence.

Rosewood oil is especially effective when added to massage oil to help combat tired muscles, especially after intense exercise.

Some herbalists use this oil to reduce the effects of migraines.

Aromatherapy Massage

Jean Valnet's work was taken up and developed by Madame Marguerite Maury, a beauty therapist who was interested in incorporating essential oils into her treatments. Her idea was to revitalize each client by using a personal aromatic blend, which she based on the individual's temperament and specific health disorders. Madame Maury was dissatisfied with the oral administration of essential oils and rediscovered the method of applying them in diluted form during massage, as had been practiced by the ancient healers.

If you would like to incorporate aromatherapy massage into your weight-management program, it is best not to use essential oils directly on your skin. They are highly concentrated and might cause a rash or skin irritation for some people. If you are

> **Cedarwood Oil (Juniperus virginiana):** If you are fearful and become easily discouraged and unmotivated during your diet, this may be the oil for you. Its dry, woodsy scent improves concentration, helps to focus scattered thoughts, and is helpful in harmonizing and focusing the mind. It is emotionally grounding and strengthening and reduces anxiety, unnecessary worries, and nervous tension. It is soothing for your fears and helpful in depression. Medical herbalists use it for its antiseptic and fungicidal properties. Good for dandruff, hair loss, dermatitis, eczema, fungal infections, and ulcers, cedarwood's sedative and grounding characteristics are also good for use in yoga or meditation.
>
> Warning: do not use during pregnancy.

going to use them through massage or through any other approach that requires absorption through the skin, it is best to dilute them with what is known as a carrier or base oil. These oils have little or no aroma of their own and are perfectly suitable for aromatherapy since they allow the essential oils themselves to work most effectively.

The best carrier oils can usually be found in health-food or natural-food stores. They will be labeled Extra Virgin or Cold Pressed. These are the first pressed oils of certain nuts, seeds, or fruits. There are hundreds of oil-bearing plants, but only a few are available commercially.

My favorite carrier oil formula is a combination of 90 percent sweet almond oil and 10 percent avocado oil. This formula is appropriate for all skin types, is good for people with dry skin, and can help relieve itching. Avocado oil is especially healing for eczema and dry dehydrated skin. You can add a little vitamin E (just puncture a capsule and squeeze it in) to keep the oil fresh and reduce rancidity.

If you keep the oil in the fridge, it may become slightly cloudy. If kept in an area that is at room temperature for a few minutes, it will become clear again.

Clary Sage Oil (Salvia sclarea): This sweet and heady oil is distilled from a flowering herb native to southern Europe and has been traditionally cultivated in the Mediterranean, Russia, the United States, England, Morocco, and central Europe. The Moroccan, French, and English sage are considered to be of the best quality for aromatherapy.

The pervading aroma of clary sage was greatly valued in the Middle Ages, but had largely fallen out of general use until the last hundred years. Sage oil has antispasmodic qualities and is an effective relaxant and sedative. In addition, the oil is antibacterial, anticonvulsive, antiseptic, an astringent, and cholesterol reducing.

When your willpower is tested or you feel run down both physically and emotionally, this sensual, nut-like scented oil is the one to choose. It is valued as a mood elevator, and its uplifting qualities may ease feelings of depression while relaxing you with a sense of euphoria. Clary sage is valuable for the treatment of tension, anxiety, and that sense of mental burnout that is common for people struggling to lose weight. The oil may also prove effective in the treatment of migraines and stress-related disorders.

It blends especially well with many other oils including pine, jasmine, lavender, bergamot, geranium, juniper, frankincense, cedarwood, and many of the citrus oils.

Warning: do not use during pregnancy.

Losing Weight through Aromatherapy

In recent years, researchers and marketers in the perfume, scent, and aroma industry have found that food-related scents and aromas can be used to help control weight. It has to do with the ways that people associate food with safety. "Mother, home, food—those words have made the industry perk up its nose," says Annette Green, chairwomen of the Sense of Smell Institute in New York. This nonprofit group provides grants for researchers studying the effects of odor on behavior. They recently conducted

Clove Oil (Syzygium aromaticum): This spicy, antiseptic oil is extracted from the buds and leaves of the plant and has traditionally been used as a muscle relaxant and soothing agent, especially for gum pain and digestive problems. It is also effective as a mosquito repellant.

Used as a breath freshener in Chinese courts, cloves were introduced into Venice by Arabian traders and distributed throughout the rest of Europe by the Venetians. Botanical researchers have defined its main constituents as eugenol, eugenyl acetate, and caryophyllene in the bud, and eugenol and eugenyl acetate in the leaves.

Cloves blend well with many other oils including basil, nutmeg, orange, black pepper, cinnamon, lemon, peppermint, rosemary, rose, citronella, and grapefruit.

Many Indian and Caribbean recipes utilize cloves in cooking dishes, especially in spiced drinks.

Warning: clove is a powerful skin irritant and should be used carefully. Do not use this oil during pregnancy.

a study that supports the assertion that food-related creams and sprays can reduce food cravings of chronic dieters. According to an article in the *New York Times* (La Ferla), "Susan Schiffman, a professor of medical psychology who specializes in eating disorders at Duke University Medical School, discovered in a study that for some people, simply inhaling can be almost as satisfying as eating." According to Professor Schiffman, "What you want sometimes is just their smell or taste, not the sensation of chewing." For example, inhaling cassia or cinnamon will help fulfill your craving for sweets.

Food-based aromas surround us. There are food-based cosmetic and skin care products everywhere. Peanut butter, cocoa butter, banana, chocolate, coffee, grape jelly, and ginger root are just a few of the foods whose aromas have been integrated into non-edible treats of one form or another because they can make us feel nurtured and energized.

> **Coffee Oil (Coffea arabica):** Coffee is an adrenal gland and nervous system stimulant, and I do not recommend drinking it as a weight-loss tool. However, the essential oil of coffee has a pleasant and stimulating aroma. Useful for improving mental clarity, uplifting for the mood, and physically energizing, I enjoy smelling the aroma of coffee grounds to start my day. I do not recommend this if you are a heavy coffee drinker and are trying to cut back or quit.

The importance of the relationship between our sense of smell and our sense of taste helps explain our interest in food-based aromas. Olfaction, our sense of smell, is actually responsible for 90 percent of what we perceive as taste. There is a physiological connection between the aroma of food and the satiety center in the brain that lets a person know when they have eaten enough. With this knowledge, we can now work safely and effectively with the body as opposed to restrictive dieting to achieve weight loss. No matter how well you eat, excessive amounts of any food may compromise your weight-control goals.

The scents we associate with food as well as the scents of herb and flower essences stimulate the limbic portion of the brain, the part that is responsible for feelings of both discomfort and well-being. It's been found that aromatherapy can actually be used as an alternative to antidepressants and tranquilizers. It can also help to balance the body during times of anxiety, which can be stressful times of weight fluctuation. A combination of calming oils, such as geranium, lavender, neroli, or sandalwood, with an uplifting oil, such as bergamot or basil, would be ideal. You can use the oils topically, in a bath, or in a light-ring burner.

In terms of eating and aromatherapy, most healthy nutritional programs relate to portion control by defining the size of a serving. Often you might have a nutritious meal without realizing that you are eating two or three servings at just one sitting. Aromatherapy can help you reduce the sizes of the

Coriander Oil (Coriandum sativum): A sensuous, sweet-smelling, spicy essence, coriander is used in massage oil blends to reduce stiffness and muscle pain. Known traditionally as an aphrodisiac, it is refreshing and stimulating in the bath. Botanical chemists have isolated its main constituents as linalol, decyl aldehyde, borneol, geraniol, carvone, and anethole.

As a food spice, coriander is used in many ethnic dishes. Coriander blends well with many other oils including cypress, neroli, orange, cinnamon, ginger, jasmine, bergamot, black pepper, citronella, galbanum, and lemon.

servings you choose in a way that doesn't leave you feeling deprived. How is that possible? According to Alan R. Hirsch, M.D., the Medical Director of the Smell & Taste Treatment & Research Foundation in Chicago, it has to do with the hypothalamus, the part of the brain where many basic drives are regulated.

The satiety center is located in the ventromedial nucleus of the hypothalamus. We stop eating when the hypothalamus signals fullness. We know this part of the brain is responsible because studies with hamsters have shown that if the ventromedial nucleus of the hypothalamus is damaged, the animal will continue to eat, non-stop, until it dies. It doesn't know when to stop eating, because it has no sense of being full.

Our olfactory bulb is connected to the satiety center of the hypothalamus. When odor molecules travel to the olfactory bulb, the brain correlates the amount of odor to the amount of food taken in. So, the satiety center uses the odor to send the message, "I've smelled it, so I must have eaten it."

As we inhale, odor molecules enter the nose. These molecules go to the pin-sized area of the olfactory membrane located just behind the bridge of the nose. Here is where the millions of olfactory receptors are found. The odor moves through a protective, mucous-coated membrane called the *epithelia* and binds to

> **Cubeb Berry Oil (Cubeba officinalis):** This spicy oil is popular among herbalists for increasing circulation, improving digestion, clearing out the sinuses and breathing passages, and relieving aches and pains. Considered an aphrodisiac in many cultures, ninth-century Arabian physicians often included cubeb berries in love potions. Today the herb is used predominantly as a culinary spice and is particularly useful in seasoning soups.

receptor sites on the olfactory nerve. These millions of receptor sites are very specific in that they are each designated to discriminate between each odor detected in our environment.

Once an odor has reached a receptor site, the body sends an electric signal to the brain via a thin, long neuron nerve cell called a *bipolar receptor cell.* Because the body sends an electrical signal, it really is sending a representation of the odor to the brain. For the brain to respond to the odor, it is intensified one thousand times its original scent. Neither hearing nor vision compare to the direct gateway the olfactory sense has to the brain.

Also, unlike other senses, the smell center is located in the emotional or limbic portion of our brains. The limbic lobe is found above the part of our brain that controls our autonomic responses (breathing, heartbeat, digestion), and below the cerebral cortex, which is the intellectual portion of the brain.

The limbic lobe is responsible for activating our hypothalamus, which in turn signals our pituitary gland to release hormones that regulate important functions in the body. The limbic lobe is also our emotional storehouse. It is here that our moods are regulated, memories are kept, and our likes and dislikes are controlled. This is why a simple odor can trigger a memory from childhood.

Neurotransmitters are multifunctional chemicals in the brain that allow nerve impulses to move from neuron to neuron. In detecting and reacting to odors, the neurons move from the olfactory bulb through the limbic lobe. Neurotransmitters are also

Cumin Seed Oil (Cuminum cyminun): The sharp, spicy aroma of this oil has made it popular for those who have mental or physical exhaustion. It is especially of value for those struggling with their weight since it had been shown to stimulate the metabolism of those who are obese.

This potent seed is an essential ingredient in curry powders as well as a basic seasoning in numerous Mexican, Indian, and Middle Eastern recipes.

Warning: it is not good to put this oil on your skin before going into the sun since it may increase photosensitivity or irritate some skins.

responsible for emotional well-being and the regulation of moods. So, here again we see the connection between emotion and our sense of smell.

The only sense that is processed in the limbic system before interpretation by the thalamus is the sense of smell. The thalamus operates as a sort of tag team with the cerebral cortex. It signals the brain about environmental changes and sensation. Take our sense of touch, for example. First, the cerebral cortex and thalamus respond by identifying a texture. This is then passed on to the limbic system, where it is decided whether you like how it feels or not. The same process is true for vision.

Smell is just the opposite; you react first, then identify. Without any logical thinking, you react to odors. This explains how we have such strong, often irrational, reactions to smell.

In understanding how smells are linked to our emotions, it is also significant to recognize the side of the brain in which smells are processed. As many people know, the left side of the brain controls logical thought and the ability to do math, etc. The right side of the brain deals more with intuition, artistic endeavors, and other functions associated with creativity. Out of all the senses, smell is the only one processed in the emotional, creative side of the brain.

> **Cypress Oil (Cupressus sempervirens):** With its lush, woody, smoky fragrance, this astringent oil refreshes, restores, and tones. Herbalists often use it as a circulatory stimulant, antispasmodic, to reduce water retention, as a natural deodorant, and for asthma. It also has a generally warming effect on the body.
>
> Most of the best cypress oil is extracted from the leaves and stems of French plants. When emotional or mental crisis looms, this oil is most effective when used in warm foot soaks. The main chemical constituents of cypress oil are pirene, sylvestrene, cymene, sabinol.
>
> This oil blends well with rosemary, sandalwood, lavender, juniper, lavender, lemon, orange, bergamot, and clary sage.

Odors are processed in the emotional center of our brains because they are necessary for our survival. Not only do we react to the smell of cut roses, or Mom's casserole, but we also respond to odors we don't consciously detect. Pheromones are odorous substances that abound in the human and animal world. It is believed that these scents were responsible for man's early survival. Through the years, our reliance on smell has been replaced with our reliance on vision. Many overweight people complain that they see food and are then hungry, when the truth really is that they detect the odor of the food and then have the conditioned response to eat or not eat, depending on whether they like the smell or not.

What we describe as smell is not just an odor, but is a combination of an odor molecule and a stimulus to another nerve found in the nose and face. This nerve, known as the trigeminal nerve, is an irritant nerve that causes the eyes to burn when we cry. It is also involved when we sneeze to help purge our systems when an irritant enters the nasal passages. It flips into action whether we cut an onion or cry from sadness.

This nerve responds to an odor whether consciously detected or not, and therefore continues to function even when a person's sense

Elemi Oil (Canarium commune): The scent of this oil helps create an environment that is conducive to meditation and introspection, and is especially helpful when inhaled when the Bach Remedies are being used. Its main constituents—phellandrene, dipentene, elemol, elemicin, terpineol, limonene, pinene—are stimulating for the immune system, and many herbalists use the oil for those recovering from a debilitating illness. Its constituents make it valuable as an expectorant and to open up the air passages. Elemi oil has been found to help the healing process of some asthmatics. An aid to those with sleeping disorders, it is valuable for weight loss in that it creates a helpful environment for those evaluating the emotional source of their overeating, especially during counseling sessions.

of smell is lost or damaged. For this reason, eating foods that stimulate the trigeminal nerve, such as peppermint, chili pepper, and horseradish, have been found to be helpful in restoring sensations.

Perhaps you've had the experience of fainting and having someone revive you with smelling salts. It happens because the trigeminal nerve is stimulated, which activates the part of the brain that keeps you awake. Tear gas also has a similar effect in that burning eyes and difficulty in breathing are responses to an odor. In both cases it is an odor that stimulates a nerve.

Did you ever hold your nose so you wouldn't have to taste something? Cough medicine, carrots, or broccoli? It seemed to work, didn't it? The same applies to all foods. If you held your nose and took a bite of the world's best chocolate, you probably wouldn't taste a thing. Because smell is more than 90 percent of taste, taste becomes a misnomer in that we really only distinguish between four different categories: bitter, salty, sweet, and sour. Beyond these, we are left with flavor.

Women become more sensitive to smells when they are ovulating. This increase in olfaction may also explain why a woman's appetite also increases during this phase.

> **Eucalyptus Oil (Eucalyptus fruticetorum):** There are many varieties of eucalyptus, but most of them are known for their antiseptic, toning, and stimulating qualities. This oil, which is generally distilled from the leaves and stems, has a camphoraceous scent that makes it popular for baths and massage during the cold season, especially in vaporizers to keep air germ-free in a sick room. Its main chemical constituents, which include cineol, pinene, limonene, cymene, phellandrene, terpinene, and aromadendrene, make it an effective deodorant, antiseptic, and soothing agent. Eucalyptus oil is a powerful, penetrating anti-viral and bacterial oil that is great for relieving respiratory infections and can also be used as an antiseptic for wounds. It has a balancing effect on the entire body.
>
> Eucalyptus blends well with thyme, pine, lavender, lemon, lemongrass, coriander, and juniper.
>
> Warning: do not use during pregnancy.
>
> **Palmarosa Oil (Cymbopogon martini):** A light floral scent that is uplifting, refreshing, and gently soothing. It promotes clarity of thought and helps all skin types, especially dry skin.

We crave variety in our diets, so it is no wonder that after a few days, people also become tired of smelling the same odor. Sweet smells tend to be our favorites. So, in using green apple, peppermint, and banana scents, it has been confirmed that odors really can help people to lose weight. In a study, the average participant lost five pounds per month using these scents to aid them, and those with a higher sensitivity to smells lost weight even more quickly.

Many of us feel hungry when we smell food. This is a learned response. Just as we have programmed ourselves to salivate when we smell doughnuts, we can unlearn or deprogram ourselves not to feel hunger at the smell of food. It is liberating to know that we can recondition ourselves to smell an odor and not just respond to

Patchouli Oil (Pogostemon patchouli): This musky, deeply sensual, and earthy oil possesses a lingering and uplifting quality that is clearing for the mind. Patchouli oil is known for preventing viral infection, healing wounds, and repelling moths.

Rose Oil (Rosa damascena): Known as the Queen of Oils, rose is among the most costly of all aromatic oils, valued throughout the centuries as having sensual and even aphrodisiacal properties. Extracted from the flowers of Bulgarian and Moroccan plants, it possesses an exquisite deep floral scent that is cooling, balancing, calming, toning, and luxurious in quality as well as in multifaceted application. Rose oil is soothing for the emotionally troubled and uplifting for those who feel sad and lack self-confidence. It tones the female reproductive system and has a sensual, romantic aspect that makes it especially popular with female dieters who are feeling uncomfortable about their bodies during the weight-loss process. Most of the rose oil available commercially is synthetic, due to the high cost of the natural product, but the actual plant-derived oil has a softness and subtlety that cannot be duplicated in a laboratory.

it by eating. With the scent disassociated from the food, hunger disappears, the desire to eat is quelled, and what is a powerful and sometimes destructive pattern is broken.

If you decide to use this program, I suggest that you commit to using an inhaler device so that you can let the tremendous power of scents assist you in losing weight. Once you start using an inhaler regularly, it becomes a habit, so you'll naturally remember to take yours with you wherever you go.

There are many reasons for the success of the inhaler devices in assisting weight loss, including the fact that they break social conditioning and change the brain chemistry. Many aromatherapists report, for instance, that any of the following oils may be used to combat depression: allspice, ambrette, basil, bergamot,

Frankincense Oil (Bosellia carterii resin): Frankincense probably has stronger religious connections historically than any other plant-derived scent. One of the most highly valued oils of the ancient world, as much as gold, it has been used since Egyptian times where it was burnt at altars as an offering to the gods. Frankincense oil is also used to aid in prayer and meditation and as a healing tool for varied health problems of the respiratory system and the genito-urinary tract. It is produced mainly in the Red Sea regions as well as in China, Somalia, South Arabia, and in smaller amounts in India. Its name is derived from the old French words *franc encens,* meaning luxuriant scent. Having a strong scent that was historically favored by both men and women, it was also used to fumigate the sick, the aim being to banish the evil spirits responsible for the illness.

Frankincense oil helps weight-management programs. It has a long-lasting, woodsy, spicy, and slightly lemony scent that serves as an aid for visualization exercises, strengthens and calms the mind, and slows the breathing while encouraging a sense of motivation, inspiration, and feelings of well-being. Its calming action is helpful for those who exhibit obsessive-compulsive patterns with food and who have painful memories that produce anxiety.

Unlike other aromatics, frankincense oil is not actually derived directly from the leaves or flowers of the plant, but rather from an oleo gum collected from a small tree or shrub with plentiful leaves and pale pink or white flowers. The oleo is harvested by making incisions in the bark. The frankincense is formed when the milky white liquid that is given off solidifies into tear-shaped amber/orange/brown lumps. The whitish gum is then dissolved and distilled to produce the essential oil. It combines well with cinnamon.

Warning: do not use during pregnancy.

Canadian balsam, cassie, cedarwood, clary sage, grapefruit, helichrysum, jasmine, lavender, Melissa, neroli, orange, patchouli, rose, rosemary, rosewood, thyme, violet, and ylang-ylang.

Fennel Seed Oil (Foeniculum vulgare): Through its primary constituents: anethole, anisic acid, anisic aldehyde, pinene, camphene, estragole, fenone, and phellandrene, herbalists have traditionally used fennel oil as an antiseptic, aphrodisiac, soothing agent, and muscle relaxant. The sweet aniseed-like aroma of this oil is also soothing for the digestive system and has historically been used to break up constipation, nausea, and abdominal gas while reducing menopausal problems. Its value in weight management occurs because it helps eliminate obesity by reducing food cravings. Fennel can also be used to help detoxify. Fennel seed oil blends well with basil, geranium, rose, rosemary, lavender, lemon, and sandalwood.

In food preparation, fennel seeds add a refreshing flavor to herb and spice blends. They can be substituted for dill and anise in many recipes, and are commonly mixed with grated coconut and served as an after-dinner snack in Indian restaurants as an aid to digestion and to counter bad breath.

Warning: fennel oil can be a skin irritant. Do not use it on young children. Do not use during pregnancy, or if you suffer from epilepsy.

As valuable as these oils are, it is important to remember that inhaler devices are contraindicated for people with asthma and those who suffer from migraine headaches. Some scents can trigger a headache, and while asthma sufferers may still use their nose to lose weight, using these devices is not advisable.

In order to maintain your interest in the program, make sure you vary the odors you use. Just as you would get tired of eating a tuna fish sandwich for every meal, you'll get tired of breathing the same odors, no matter how good they smell in the beginning.

Remember: these oils are very concentrated. They should never be used internally as part of this weight-management program. Some oils may cause photosensitivity and should not be employed before exposure to the sun. Some oils should not be used during pregnancy.

> **Melissa Oil (Melissa officinalis):** Commonly known as Lemon Balm, this sharp, lemony, floral-scented oil has a soothing and at the same time uplifting effect on mind and body. This is especially true when used in the bath (just two or three drops of the oil in a full tub is all that is required). Its primary constituents are citronellal, geraniol, citral, linalyl acetate, and eugenol. It is a comforting oil during times when the pollen count is very high and during the winter months.
>
> Dilute to 1 percent and use only three drops in a bath as it may cause irritation.
>
> Warning: do not use Melissa oil on the skin in direct sunlight.

Aromatherapy and Breathing Exercise

1. Stand with your feet six inches apart.
2. Clasp your fingers together in front of you and let your arms relax.
3. Inhale deeply while you bring your clasped hands straight over your head. (As the arms move up on the inhalation, imagine them floating on the breath.)
4. Let your forearms fall behind your head.
5. Place a little pressure on the heels of your hands, and start your exhalation as your arms return to where they began in front of you.
6. Now inhale your aromatic oil of choice.
7. Pause and hold the breath to the count of three.
8. Exhale the aroma slowly.
9. Repeat this cycle ten times, inhaling the aroma with each cycle.

A Word about Displacement

Many people who quit smoking start to chew gum to curb their desire for a cigarette. Substituting one behavior with another is called displacement. The inhalers work by displacing the urge to eat with smelling scents.

Geranium Oil (Pelargonium odoratissimum): This oil is extracted by steam distillation from the leaves and stems of plants native to South Africa and is widely cultivated in Egypt, Russia, and China. The sweet, floral, rose-like scent of this oil may help one achieve an overall feeling of tranquillity, emotional security, and well-being. The main constituents of geranium oil are geraniol, borneol, termineol, limonene, phellandrene, pinene, citronellal, and linalol.

Therapeutically, the oil is inhaled for its influence on the emotions and nervous system and its influence in reducing the body's response to physical stress. Geranium oil is calming, balancing, and uplifting, and is useful for depression, nervous tension, and anxiety. Geranium oil is often mixed with sweet almond oil for massage, especially where there is cellulite and for the treatment of psoriasis and eczema.

Geranium blends well with rosemary, sandalwood, cedarwood, citronella, clary sage, lavender, lime, neroli, orange, lavender, bergamot, petit grain, grapefruit, jasmine, rose citrus oils, and any floral oils.

Warning: do not use during pregnancy.

Displacement does not signify a weakness in any way. It is simply the replacement of one behavior with another. As humans, we eat when there is food available because of our evolutionary past. Early humans didn't have a regular supply of food, so they ate when there was food at hand. Using displacement is nothing to be ashamed of. Rather, it is something to celebrate in that it shows that you have made a decision to improve your life.

Inhalers work in the sense that their presence is a reminder to use them as a substitute for eating. Most reminders work within the cognitive or intellectual left side of the brain. For example, when you find yourself wanting to nibble, you see your inhaler and your brain sends the message "I'm not hungry," or

> **Goldenrod Oil (Solidago canadensis):** This introspective oil is encouraging for those who do not communicate their needs easily. It also promotes an interest in meditation.

"I just ate," thereby curbing the urge to eat. The inhaler device actually stimulates your brain to override the emotional urges to eat.

Some people worry about replacing the habit of overeating with over-sniffing from the inhaler, but inhaling is harmless and is a much better alternative to overeating. As you continue to use the inhaling devices, you'll begin to notice the times that you have cravings. Inhaling is very helpful not only in reducing the intake of food, but also in creating insight into lifetime behavioral patterns that have led you to overeating. Once you know your patterns, you can change them.

Our emotions often rule our behavior, so it is possible that odor devices work to control food cravings because they reduce frustration, and therefore give an overall sense of well-being.

It's true that those who have a good sense of smell lose weight faster than those who do not. However, with the exception of those who suffer from no ability to smell, the use of an inhaler can work for anyone.

You may want to keep a journal of your progress. Some people find it helpful to log in such items as what they eat on a given day and how the device helped in curbing their cravings. If used regularly, the inhalers will definitely work.

Also, to assist you in using aromas along with your diet, make sure that you take the time to actually smell your food before you eat it. The scent will travel to your olfactory bulb in the brain and stimulate the satiety center. This simple action will help you eat less at each meal. And be sure to chew your food well. You've heard that chewing your food aids digestion. But each time you chew, you also release more of the food's odor, and your body thinks that it is ingesting more than it actually is.

> **Grapefruit Oil (Citrus paradisi):** This lovely, fresh, clear, citrus-scented oil is derived by crushing grapefruit skins. Grapefruit oil is refreshing and reviving for the mind and emotions. Its main constituents are limonene, paradisiol, neral, geraniol, and citronellal. These make it a digestive stimulant, lymphatic stimulant, balancing for nervous exhaustion, and helpful for reducing water retention. Grapefruit blends well with bergamot, orange, and other citrus oils.
>
> Warning: grapefruit oil may cause photosensitivity; do not use before exposure to the sun. Do not use this oil during pregnancy.

Aromatherapy Tips for Your Food Choices

Many of us will admit to having a sweet tooth. Scientists have found that craving sweets may actually be our body's way of trying to boost our chemical levels. The group of neurotransmitters linked with sweet cravings is called serotonin, and serotonin has been linked to happiness.

There are drugs (i.e., Fen-Phen) that increase serotonin and therefore reduce cravings and appetite. There are also drugs (i.e., Prozac) that are serotonin agonists, which increase the level of serotonin in the body. Many people take Prozac for treatment of depression and as a side effect find that their appetite and craving for sweets is reduced, even if they aren't trying to lose weight. It is also thought that because chemicals work in chains (one is produced to stimulate the production of another chemical), craving certain foods such as chocolate may be our body's way of stimulating the production of the neurotransmitter of chocolate. So, sometimes you may really need chocolate.

Stress, frustration, depression, and PMS often increase our desire for comfort foods. We eat to medicate our moods. Since taste is 90 percent smell, it is possible to sniff the cravings away. The smell of chocolate alone increases the body's production of serotonin, for example. Frustration is reduced by smelling the odor because that satisfies the craving.

Lime Oil (Citrus aurantifolia): This energizing, uplifting oil is wonderful when added to bath water (just a few drops). Generally produced from the peels of West Indian fruits, lime oil acts much like lemon oil and other citrus oils. This sweet oil is the one of choice if you are recovering from a major illness. Lime oil blends well with citronella, rosemary, lavender, lavandin, clary sage, and neroli.

Jasmine Oil (Absolute jasminum officinale): Jasmine is a very costly oil. The jasmine generally grown for its oil is found in Egypt. This floral-scented oil requires a vast quantity of blossoms, which must be gathered at night when the scent is at its highest in order to produce a few drops of oil. When in a state of self-doubt, this heady, emotionally warming, exotic perfume raises the spirits and soothes, uplifts, nurtures, and boosts self-confidence. Just a few drops of jasmine are good for reducing stress and general anxiety. Herbalists have used jasmine oil as an antiseptic and a soothing agent for the skin. Its sensual qualities have made it popular in some cultures as an aphrodisiac.

When a person is tired or frustrated, cravings are usually at their peak. Restrictive dieting increases frustration, therefore increasing cravings. It is craving that usually starts the rebound pattern in dieting. No one is sure of the exact mechanisms that are responsible for cravings. More research into brain chemistry will probably give us the answer one day. What is helpful in alleviating cravings is eating a variety of foods, eating regularly, getting lots of rest, and using those scents and aromas that will reduce your desire to eat sweets.

Among the herbs that will serve you best in this area are the scents of nutmeg, allspice, and cocoa butter. You may also want to use the herb-based sweetener Stevia.

Another way to reduce your cravings for sweets is to choose foods throughout the day that have prominent tastes and aromas.

Eating these small amounts of different aromatic foods is also quite advantageous to those who want to lose weight. The Japanese do this quite well, whereas Americans typically use large portions of one food.

Choose foods that are hot or spicy to the taste. Hot food not only is better for your digestion, but also naturally releases the odors of the food you eat. People generally eat less of a meal when they have a cup of hot soup as an appetizer.

Eating spicy or strong-flavored foods also helps people lose weight more quickly. We consume too many bland foods because we are a society on the run. Even when you do have to eat plain foods, such as bagels or popcorn, choose a flavored variety.

Try to avoid dairy foods when you are trying to lose weight. There are a number of reasons for this. One is the bland taste and the other is lack of aroma. Since our satiety center is not triggered by milk odor molecules, we may have the tendency to overconsume them in a way that we would not overconsume foods with a stronger taste or aroma.

Aromatherapy and Mood Disorders

Research has shown that tastes and odors help us cope emotionally. People who lose their sense of smell are much more likely to develop generalized anxiety disorders (Noell). One theory holds that subliminal smells exist that are capable of influencing human behavior. Those who have lost their sense of smell may not benefit from the subliminal scents that seem to be an integral part of mood regulation.

Since smell is linked so heavily to emotions, odors, in the form of aromatherapy, are now being used to treat mood disorders. The scent of jasmine, for example, stimulates changes in the front of the brain, causing us to be more alert. The scent of lavender affects the back of the brain, producing a more relaxed state. Consequently, sufferers of insomnia may benefit from a few drops of lavender on their pillows to induce a more restful sleep. A sniff of jasmine in the morning can be a substitute for caffeine.

> **Ylang-Ylang (Cananga odorata):** Useful as an aphrodisiac, the floral aroma of this emotionally uplifting and physically relaxing oil has a regulating effect on an overstimulated nervous system. This makes it valuable as an antidepressant and sedative. Ylang-Ylang is calming, euphoric, and effective for treating hypertension, depression, stress, insomnia, tension, anger, and the frustration often associated with obesity.

Other scents that have been tested successfully for mood disorders include green apple and cucumber for claustrophobia, and vanilla, nutmeg, and apple for various forms of anxiety. Aside from reducing the appetite, food odors have also been found useful in relieving frustration. Because a pleasant odor can remind a person of a childhood memory of happy times, odors reduce frustration. Food aromas can help you reduce weight because they reduce the frustration that leads to cravings. Since tastes and odors help us to cope emotionally, it is clear that we can employ them as tools for losing weight.

The most effective scents are derived from complete, whole botanical distillates or expressions, such as vanilla, cocoa butter, and cinnamon. These "natural" oils have not been extracted with chemical solvents, nor are they synthetic fragrance oils. Most fruit- or food-related scents have been enhanced with synthetic additives in order to create a "banana" or "candy" scent that smells more like the actual food than the food itself. Pure oils are best when aromatherapy is being used for purely therapeutic purposes, since they are the concentrated molecular constituents that give a botanical its fragrance. Plant-derived essential oils are an extension and a reflection of the "life force" of a plant, and might even be to a plant what hormones are to humans. You may find it beneficial, however, to use scents that are designed to imitate the aroma of food, since they can help reduce food cravings.

The use of stimulating odors such as peppermint or jasmine may also work to reduce frustration and overeating. A problem is

Sandalwood (Santalum album): This oil has traditionally been burned as an aid to meditation and has been used in religious ceremonies. Also employed as a body fragrance, this persistent, exotic, rich, and musky oil is popular for relieving tension and for creating a sense of calm and grounding for both the body and mind. Generally extracted by steam distillation from the woody portion of sandalwood trees in East India, its main constituents are forneol, santalone, santalols, and fusanols. It is an ideal remedy for reducing nervous depression, fear, and stress, and has been used traditionally as an aphrodisiac. As a tool for weight loss, this oil is most effective when used with visualization exercises throughout the day.

Sandalwood oil blends well with jasmine, clove, lavender, black pepper, bergamot, rose, violet, geranium, labdanum, vetiver, patchouli, mimosa, and myrrh.

Peppermint (Mentha piperita): One of the most important and popular herbs in the world is peppermint. Its energizing menthol fragrance has an intensely penetrating and stimulating quality. Usually derived by steam distillation from plants grown in the United States, its main constituents include thymol, pinene, cineol, limonene, menthone, and menthol.

Peppermint oil is highly effective in reducing digestive upset, nausea, headaches, coughs, poor circulation (especially in tired feet), mental and physical fatigue, muscular pains, and sinus congestion, and has a calming effect on the emotions without the sedating quality associated with other calming oils.

Peppermint oil is stimulating, refreshing, cooling, restorative, and uplifting to mind and body. It can be added to a massage oil blend to help stimulate the digestive system and blends well with rosemary and juniper, especially in the bath. Other oils that peppermint blends well with include sandalwood, lavender, marjoram, bergamot, geranium, and rosemary.

usually magnified tenfold when a person is tired. Odors that help you to stay alert make it easier for the cerebral cortex to inhibit impulsive drives such as overeating. These scents don't have to be used in an inhaler. Potpourri mixtures, scented candles, room sprays, and vials of scents sold in specialty stores can be used in your home or office.

Another strategy for weight loss is to avoid alcohol before and with your meal. Alcohol inhibits the cerebral cortex, which is responsible for rational and logical thoughts, allowing the limbic portion of the brain to take control.

Let me emphasize here that restrictive dieting is the worst enemy for someone who wants to lose weight. To begin to lose weight, eat regular meals and start to make use of inhaling aromas. As you continue to use the odors, you'll notice that your helpings get smaller. Once you start to lose weight, think about ways to make your favorite meals with less fat, sugar, and salt. Foods that are low-fat, low-sugar, and low-salt are not only healthy but can be delicious and emotionally satisfying. A great way to integrate aromatherapy into your herbal weight-loss program is through mental imagery, also known as self-hypnosis or visualization.

Visualization Techniques and Aromatherapy

Your self-image plays an important role in weight loss. Try to visualize yourself in two distinct pictures: one is the "before" picture, or the overweight you; the other is the "after" picture, or the new, slimmer you. Use the "before" picture to convince yourself of the need to lose weight. Use the "after" picture to keep your goal in mind and for continued encouragement and motivation.

Try this visualization technique. Find a quiet place where you will not be disturbed. Sit in a straight-backed chair with both feet on the floor and hold your hands, palms up, on your knees. Close your eyes. Inhale and exhale the recommended oil deeply and slowly. As you exhale, visualize your "after" picture, and see what you will look like after you have reached your weight-loss goals.

Complete your visualization by 1) taking a long, deep breath of the aromatic oil, 2) slowly exhaling, and 3) gradually opening your eyes. Sit quietly for a few minutes, as you become aware once again of your surroundings. Slowly begin to wiggle your fingers and toes. Rise only after you feel acclimated to your surroundings.

Typically, people who lose weight successfully tend to maintain weight loss when they have tailored the program to their own personal favorite foods, time schedules, and quirks. First, make a list of all of your favorite foods. Then, inhale the aromatic oil of, let's say, strawberries, three times while using the visualization program described below. Even as you apply aromatherapy, you may occasionally feel deprived as you remember your old eating patterns. When this happens, it is essential that you avoid sabotaging your eating program through bingeing. For this reason, it's best to avoid drastic calorie reductions as you begin the program. Extreme caloric reductions make it more difficult for you to lose fat by lowering your metabolic rate and reducing the rate at which your body burns calories.

After you have eliminated the foods that will not support your weight control goals, start to integrate those that you are fond of into the thirty-day meal structure described in Part Two of this book.

Aroma-Assisted Visualization

1. Find a place to sit quietly without interruption for a few minutes.
2. Prepare a diffusion of essential oil. You might use jasmine, lavender, sandalwood, or a combination of these. Put three or four drops on a tissue and place the tissue near your nose, either on a nearby table or shelf or tucked into the neck of your shirt. Or, if you have the space and time, use an essential oil diffuser.
3. Sit erect but relaxed, preferably in a chair with a firm, straight back. Planted solidly upright in this chair, with your feet flat on the floor, rest your hands on your lap or thighs with the palms turned upward.

> **Rosemary Oil (Rosmarinus officinalis):** The warm, refreshing, invigorating, woody scent of this oil is a powerful mental stimulant that aids concentration. It is generally extracted by stream distillation from Tunisian plants. It is particularly of value when you are feeling "burned out." The Latin name *Rosmarinus* means "dew of the sea." And the oil of this "dew" has an uplifting toning effect on the emotions that makes it a popular scent for those experiencing mental fatigue, depression, and poor memory. For those who yo-yo diet, rosemary oil is valuable in that it helps focus concentration and helps bring the individual back to their original intention.
>
> Valuable in relieving the joint stiffness that can plague obese individuals with osteo-arthritis, rosemary oil also helps relieve water retention. The main constituents in rosemary oil are cineol, lineol, borneol, camphene, pinene, camphor, and terpineol. This oil blends well with olibanum, citronella, thyme, elemi, cedarwood, lavender, lavandin, basil, peppermint, labdanum, petit grain, and cinnamon.
>
> Warning: do not use this oil if you are pregnant, suffering from high blood pressure, or have epilepsy.

4. Close your eyes and turn all your attention to your breath. Breathe in deeply and very slowly.
5. Form two images, one as you exhale and the other as you inhale. As you exhale, visualize sticky ooze slowly draining throughout your body, into a central canal, then down through both legs and out the bottoms of the feet. Take a good look at this ooze. You see that it is composed of innumerable toxins carried in a vehicle of semi-liquid fat. As you inhale, allow the image to disappear and replace it with the light or color from the aroma.
6. When you have performed this exercise for five to fifteen minutes, take a very long deep breath and exhale even more slowly, opening your eyes very gradually. Do not

move your eyes for a few moments, but merely take in your surrounds without purposely looking at anything.

7. After a while, move your toes and fingers, then slowly get up and return to whatever you were doing before sitting down.

Chapter 6

Flower Remedies

It would not be inaccurate to say that a spiritual hunger combined with emotional stress is a major cause of obesity and other eating disorders, including anorexia, bulimia, and related illnesses. Our society has deified thinness and has promoted it constantly through television, radio, print media, and the fashion culture. This constant selling of the idea that a sense of salvation—happiness, contentment, and a more meaningful life—comes with an ideal body has caused both men and women to become obsessed with food and thinness. Many people restrict their caloric intake to dangerously low levels, and then binge from an emotional need to gain a sense of control and meaning in life.

Many people react to stress, tension, and the grief that comes with a great loss by overeating as well. If you are to be successful in losing weight, and maintaining a normal, healthy weight through a well-balanced herbal and dietary program, you must address the cause of your tension. You must learn to control your responses to stress, rather than become a victim of unpleasant situations. Homeopathy is one system for doing this. Dr. Edwin Bach, British scientist and physician, took the energetic principles and applied them to balancing emotional states through homeopathically prepared flower remedies. He discovered that behind many of his patient's physical ailments were certain emotional and psychological disturbances to which those illnesses were directly and undeniably linked.

Today, this may seem an obvious conclusion since, in the current Age of Information, psychology is uncontested as a science. One need only log on to their personal computer in order to receive therapeutic advice, free counseling, or a quick consultation with fate. But it was not so long ago that science and psychology, which was considered more emotional than rational and therefore less serious and less favorable, were so different in their makeup that they repelled one another.

Though Bach was primarily a pathologist, immunologist, and bacteriologist, he realized that inherent to these sciences was a vibrational and emotive element. By looking beyond the conventional boundaries of medical science, he was able to monitor his patients' progress from less of a distance. He took into account how they actually felt, as opposed to simply examining the symptoms exhibited in relation to particular maladies, and in doing so bridged the gap between physical and emotional pain. He also brought into question the cause and effect relationship of pain when dealing with illness.

Bach remarked in his findings that emotional problems, especially feelings of despair, hopelessness, worry, resentment, anxiety, fear, and lack of self-confidence, so depleted a patient's vitality that the body lost its natural resistance and became susceptible to a host of organic illnesses.

Today, research in such fields as psychoneuroimmunology supports these findings, not only linking the two elements of science and psychology, which had previously repelled one another like oil and vinegar, but whipping them into a holistic salad dressing, so to speak, with one ingredient indistinguishable from the other.

Today one would be hard-pressed to find a scientist or doctor who did not at least look into the emotional and psychological factors affecting a patient when attempting to cure a disease, promote weight loss or longevity, or even heal a sprained ankle or a scraped knee.

Following extensive research, Bach found that picking certain species of wild flowers at certain times in the blooming cycle, and preparing them homeopathically, optimized the healing qualities of those plants. He eliminated from his studies plants that he found to be toxic or that produced side effects. Ultimately, he succeeded in discovering thirty-eight flowering plants, trees, and special waters that had profound effects on stabilizing a wide range of mental and emotional stresses as well as dysfunctional behavior patterns.

These flower remedies were therefore indirectly effective in the treatment of physical illness. Unlike chemical drugs, which can be suppressive and can create dependencies, the Bach Remedies, as they are known today, are considered safe and non-habit forming and work by gently reestablishing emotional and psychological equilibrium. They can be used to address emotional and behavioral issues that hide behind an ailing or unsatisfactory physical façade. While other approaches might attempt to heal the behavior or emotional problems of an individual, Bach Remedies go to the person's energy source.

Considered a major healing breakthrough, these preparations have been used for more than fifty years by a broad spectrum of health-care professionals worldwide, including medical doctors, dentists, chiropractors, and psychologists, as well as the general public.

Bach Remedies are a most effective element in an herbal-based weight-management program because they address many of the subtle emotional factors that cause people to overeat. They are available in most natural food stores and are easily prepared by adding a few drops into spring water.

As you address emotional issues tied to food, you will notice that your appetite will decrease almost immediately and that there are many other more subtle benefits. You are no longer hungry all the time as you would be on many other low-calorie weight-loss schemes, and you feel mentally alive without a sense of guilt or shame.

Using Bach Remedies for Weight Management

Pick the remedy you are going to use and place two drops in a small glass of water and sip at intervals throughout the day or

> **Agrimony:** This Bach Remedy is helpful for those feel unloved but who smile in order to hide their pain from others so they won't be a burden. Many overweight people will continue to smile even when they are distressed and unable to communicate their pain. Later, they will eat in order to escape from their bottled-up troubles. Eating only causes more distress, and yet they will continue to smile, and then eat, continuing the cycle.

until relief is obtained. Replenish as necessary. For long-term use, add two drops to a thirty ml dropper bottle, top up with spring (not distilled or filtered) water, and take four drops from this solution four times daily, or more frequently if necessary, until relief is obtained. Up to six or seven remedies may be taken together if required.

If your mood changes often, or if you are bingeing or yo-yo dieting, take one dose, but if you've been feeling balanced for some time, there is no set limit as to how long you can take your chosen remedy or remedies. You cannot overdose or hurt yourself from long-term use of the Bach Remedies.

Bach Remedies are available at many natural food and health food markets. If you have difficulty obtaining them, contact the international distributor by email at info@nelsonbach.com, or call (800) 319-9151. You can also contact them by mail at:

Nelson Bach USA, Ltd
100 Research Drive
Wilmington, MA 01887

Because they are energetically based, the Bach Remedies offer a spiritual dimension to your herbal weight-loss program. The remedies create a system for bolstering faith and hope.

Dr. Bach's system was based on the concept that everyone deserves love and that there is a power greater than ourselves that will help us to restore love and sanity in our lives.

> **Aspen:** This Bach Remedy is valuable for anxious individuals who experience fear and apprehension without clear reasons. Aspen dispels tension, aids in relaxation, and is much more effective than eating food in order to relax.

Many of us fear change. Fitting into a new emotional skin can seem too difficult, too uncomfortable, or too risky to handle. You may feel that you can't go back and you can't move forward, and in this way you begin to lose hope and faith in ever breaking out of this cycle, and you may sink into despair and depression.

When you seem to have no willpower left and you begin to ask questions about whether or not this diet is worth it, Bach Remedies offer a way out of this negative type of thinking.

The remedies will help you to be honest about the reality of your life. They will help you to:
- Express your feelings
- Be honest with yourself about what makes you mad, glad, sad, etc.
- Release tension, anger, and sadness in healthy ways
- Strengthen your focus on healthy eating when you are angry about something
- If you are anxious and upset, even if there is no definable reason, the remedies can help you feel more emotionally balanced so that you do not eat the first thing within reach. The remedies can support you in dealing with rage without repressing it.

In order to use herbs and flower remedies effectively as part of your weight-management program, it is essential to integrate a stress-management program with your choice of remedies. In this way you will fill all of the emotional spaces you used to stuff with food with an understanding of the role that unresolved stress plays in overeating and weight issues.

> **Beech:** This Bach Remedy is balancing for perfectionists who tend to find fault in just about everything and everyone. People who are critical and who overreact to small annoyances or idiosyncrasies in others will benefit from this remedy and will experience greater fulfillment by limiting their opportunities for disappointment.

Understanding Stress

Stress is generally defined as a mentally and emotionally disruptive influence. Though there are positive types of stress such as sex and laughter, most people tend to think of stress in terms of its negative effects.

Of all of the body's systems, the nervous system is probably the most fragile and easily affected by stress. The delicate balance of your nervous system is taxed by a combination of emotional, physical, and chemical factors (including food allergies, sensitivity reactions, poor diet, poor water, air pollution, and noise). Stress may also appear as a response to pregnancy, family or job-related problems, a major physical trauma, or a personality type that is overly self-critical and has unreasonable expectations of others.

As a result of stress, you may suffer from a host of disorders including insomnia, nervous tension, reduced circulation, aches and pains, certain types of arthritis, alcoholism, asthma, backache, canker sores, headaches, hypertension, sexual problems, mood swings, lethargy, reduced immunological function, insomnia, dermatitis and other skin disorders, colitis, and ulcers and other gastrointestinal disorders.

Although it would be both impractical and impossible to eliminate all forms of stress and tension, there are numerous herbal approaches that we can take to minimize their effects, and the Bach Remedies are among the most useful.

Do You Overeat to Compensate for High Stress?

Many people use food to soothe their emotions and to compensate for excess tension. Are you one of these individuals? There are a

Centaury: This Bach Remedy is balancing for introverts who are overeager to please others, regardless of their own feelings and needs. Frequently weak-willed, they are easily exploited and dominated. Their own interests are often ignored or left for later and then never addressed. In order to fill those empty spaces of need, often mistaken for hunger, they will binge, which can lead to obesity. These people will be left unsatisfied, and the feeling of dissatisfaction will continue to grow as they continue to ignore their real needs. In an attempt to compensate for their neediness, they aim to please others, but their aim is off center. Centaury helps target a person's needs, thereby eliminating the process of attempting to fill a spiritual/emotional emptiness with foods that contain no nutritional value.

Cerato: This Bach Remedy is valuable for individuals who lack confidence in their own decisions and judgements. These people are constantly seeking the advice of others, leaving open the possibility for misguidance, which often occurs. Lack of confidence in oneself is detrimental when attempting to make and stick with the decision to lose weight.

number of signs that a person can evaluate to determine whether or not they are prone to obesity through stress.

These include the following:

- You eat, move about, and walk rapidly.
- You are impatient.
- You speak quickly and speed through the ends of your sentences, often speaking without sentence structure.
- You are unable to relax without feeling guilty about not working or taking care of some "important business," even on vacation.
- You usually attempt to do two or more things at the same time, for example, working while eating breakfast.
- You are extremely shy and have difficulty communicating

your needs. When confronted with an important choice in social situations, you will go with the decisions of others even to your own detriment so long as you can avoid conflict by doing so.

- You think that time management means doing more things in less time.
- You define success by how fast things are accomplished.
- You are compulsive about owning things or controlling things rather than enjoying them.

Stress Can Be Beneficial and Harmful

Although many people assume that stress is negative, this is not always the case. A certain amount of stress and tension are necessary, and are actually important in living a balanced and productive life. It is how you respond to stress that is the key. There are many ways to respond to stress that do not involve food.

Too much stress overloads the body's resources and can prove very harmful. If the body cannot handle the stress overload, it may reach a state of "pathological" tension or extreme stress. When this stress increases, your breathing may become shallow, which has a pronounced effect on the blood circulation throughout the body and reduces the amount of oxygen that reaches the brain. Stress at this level may even lead to a feeling of terror, extreme mood swings, and even emotional breakdowns.

In addition to shallow breathing, your muscles will tighten up, especially around your pelvis, neck, and shoulders. As a quick fix to reduce this tension, you may reach for high-calorie snacks and high-fat foods. Be aware that it is not only obesity that can result from excessive stress.

Understanding Your Emotions

According to some psychologists, we experience four basic emotions: happiness, sadness, fear, and joy. The level of success that you have in your weight-management program is greatly dependent on how you respond to one or another of these feelings.

Cherry Plum: This Bach Remedy is valuable for the fear of losing mental and physical control or of doing something desperate. People who experience this type of fear may have impulses to do things known or thought to be wrong.

Chestnut Bud: This Bach Remedy is recommended for people who fail to learn from experience, repeating the same pattern or mistakes again and again. This remedy is especially helpful for those with a history of yo-yo dieting.

Repressed feelings can cause you to eat more. To avoid overeating, it is essential that you learn to express how you feel, and Bach Remedies can assist you in doing that.

Emotional repression creates stress. Maybe you are fearful that if you reveal your feelings in one situation, you will be unable to control them in another. But in fact, if you do not deal with your feelings, then your underlying frustration may come out in the form of various unproductive and dysfunctional behavior patterns, including denial that you even have a weight problem and compulsive overeating. These patterns can lead to various types of physical and emotional stress.

Anger, Fear, and Stress

Of the four basic emotions, the two that seem to be the greatest roadblocks to effective weight management are anger and fear.

The way that you can obtain freedom from fear is to participate more actively in life. Some people choose to be spectators and let life pass them by. Bach Remedies will broaden your perspective so that you will be more open to experience those things that will dissipate fear and anger.

If you are serious about creating joy and freedom from fear, then consider applying some or all of the following suggestions:

- Get involved in small group activities and service organizations. By supporting other people, you are in a

Chicory: This Bach Remedy is valuable for people who experience the need to control or direct those close to them. The need to control can lead to overeating.

Clematis: This is the Bach Remedy for people who have little concern for the present and live with their heads in the clouds. Often times, overweight individuals do not pay attention to their present food consumption. They will plan to cut fat and sugar from their diet, even while eating a hamburger and soda pop.

sense helping them go beyond the limitations of fear. In this way, you learn about the importance of support as part of the process of self-actualization.

- Become involved with friends and family. Ask them for support when you require it, and don't be afraid to offer to support them emotionally when they are in need.
- Choose your circumstances and environment for work and play consciously. A creative work environment is key to success.
- Expand your interests, try new things, and avoid doing things merely out of habit. In this way, you can see life from a different perspective and make new friends and acquaintances in the process. The more expansive you are, the more you partake in and experience the joy of life.
- Bring humor into your life. Spend time with people who love to laugh, read humorous books, and listen to humorous records and tapes. Don't look at everything from such a serious perspective. In other words, lighten up.
- Look at the things in your life that you have to be grateful for. If something unpleasant comes along, don't allow fear to paralyze you. Change takes effort and skill. See this new opportunity as a new way of applying your skills. If your initial attempts do not succeed, try to create new ways to adjust. See each situation as a challenge or game to be

played, not as something that causes you to become fearful or paralyzed.

- See all situations as gifts to be used for gaining new knowledge and skills for making effective choices. Not all situations will bring ease or comfort. Making the right choice sometimes requires learning to choose in new ways than you have chosen in the past.
- Express your feelings freely whenever possible. When you hold in your feelings, the result may be that you will begin to experience a sense of hopelessness, powerlessness, and frustration. Share your feelings with friends, loved ones, or in a support group setting.
- Be patient, tolerant, and compassionate.
- Take care of a pet. The responsibility of caring for a pet and the unconditional love that animals, particularly dogs, offer their masters has been found to be a powerful tool for individuals who are isolated, out of touch with their emotions, and who feel unloved.

Stress-Reducing Exercises

Concerning weight management, the goal of using Bach Remedies is to help you to understand the underlying cause of your anxiety and overcome it. Many herbal practitioners and physicians report that Bach Remedies can be effective in treating chronic, moderate anxiety states as well as simple phobias. In subtle ways, these remedies can assist a person in modifying eating patterns. This may be done without necessarily addressing the underlying causes of fear and anxiety. I have personally found this technique to be effective when combined with a variation of an approach known as systemic desensitization. In our approach, the client is taught a stress-reducing technique in which they visualize eating a fulfilling meal while passing over high-fat or other foods that are best avoided.

Even if you are a high-stress person, there are ways to reduce the impact of stress that enable you to be as effective as possible. I

> **Crab Apple:** This Bach Remedy is useful for individuals who suffer from low self-esteem and are constantly fearful of being contaminated. These individuals are often excessively concerned with personal cleanliness. When an individual is overweight they often have low self-esteem. It is important to raise self-esteem while losing weight.
>
> **Elm:** This Bach Remedy helps to ease painful feelings of inadequacy and being overwhelmed with responsibility—feelings that can lead an individual toward eating too much.

recommend that you practice these stress-reducing tips on a regular basis. By doing so you will be healthier, both physically and emotionally, and more effective in making conscious choices. Here are some exercises to help you relax your body and your mind:

1. Clench your fists as tightly as possible for about five seconds and then release them. Now shake your hands loosely.
2. With your head still and your eyes focused straight ahead, raise and lower your eyebrows as quickly as possible. (This will relieve forehead tension and headaches.)
3. Open your eyes as wide as you can and then squeeze them together tightly. Repeat this three or four times. Do it throughout the day to relieve eye stress and tension.
4. For range of motion of the arms, stretch and move your arms, legs, and head. These stretching exercises will give you a feeling of lightness and reduce stiffness throughout your body.
5. Develop a regular exercise program that you use at least three times a week. A good way to begin is by walking briskly or swimming laps for half an hour three times a week. For indoor aerobic exercise, use one of the exercise video tapes available or use a rebounding apparatus (a trampoline-type unit).

Gentian: This Bach Remedy helps an individual to alleviate self-doubt and discouragement. If you want to lose weight, it's important to believe in yourself and not get discouraged.

6. To release emotional frustration, use your bed or a thick pillow for the following exercise: raise both of your arms over your head with your fists tightly clenched. Hit the bed or pillow with your forearms and fists at the same time. Continue banging on the soft surface until you feel a sense of release, which you may experience as exhilaration or exhaustion.

Master the Art of Journal Writing
Write about your feelings, especially the ones you are unable to express to others. Describe them or write poems about them. The more you are able to express how you feel, the less these feelings will control you. They will be what they should be—a part of your healthy emotional makeup. The ability to express your emotions in a healthy and effective way is a sign of maturity.

Read Self-Help, Motivational, and Spiritual Books Daily
These books can help motivate, inform, and inspire you. They can help you define the self that is loving and nurturing with a clear profundity.

Surround Yourself with the Good Life
The "good life" finds a balance among pleasure, positive moods, spiritual fulfillment, and having good friends. Knowing how to live the good life is critical to psychological and physical health.

Create Time for Yourself Daily
We all need time to be alone, to think, dream, and wonder. Before you schedule time for anything else, be sure to schedule time for yourself.

Gorse: This Bach Remedy is for feelings of hopelessness and futility where there is little hope of relief. When a person is in this state they may binge or go off their weight-loss program. Gorse helps them to remember that there is a light at the end of the tunnel and helps them stay focused on their healthy weight-loss goals.

Heather: This Bach Remedy is helpful for those who seek companionship from anyone who will listen to their problems and those who have difficulty being alone. Such traits can lead to overeating.

Pleasure and positive moods are critical to psychological and physical health because psychological and emotional states affect immune function. Positive moods and happiness have beneficial health effects. We can learn to control our moods and increase our happiness. Money doesn't increase happiness, but small daily pleasures do. Tell yourself a positive story to improve your self-worth and well-being.

Share Your Feelings
Confession is not only good for the soul, it's also good for the body. Confiding in diaries or to a close friend may not only make you feel good, it may improve your health. Humans need each other. The healing power of families and friends are demonstrated to us in our everyday lives. Touch, communication, and psychological support are important factors in good health. Learn how the pleasures of company can enhance your sense of self and well-being.

Contribute to the Happiness of Others
Each of us wants to know that we make a difference in the world. No matter who you are or what your problems may be, there is always something that you can do to help others who need support. Even if you are in the depths of depression, know that there may be some small thing that you can do. Inspire ordinary people to do extraordinary things, every day.

Holly: This Bach Remedy is for those who experience feelings of suspicion, revenge, envy, and jealousy out of the need for love, feelings that can also lead to overeating.

Honeysuckle: This Bach Remedy helps free a person from obsessing about past regrets and brings them back to the present. Sometimes when people gain a lot of weight, they reminisce about a time in the past when they were thin rather then focus on creating a healthy eating program in the present.

Remember, Life Is a School, Not Just a Playground

One of the things that people must know in order to be happy is that we are here on this planet to learn—life is a kind of boot camp. You can have a very full and happy life once you accept this fact. If you resist the idea, you may spend your life struggling to find constant happiness at the end of some imaginary rainbow.

Learn to Relax

Relaxing is a healthy pleasure in itself, and you need it to live life to the fullest. Simple ways to relax include meditation, prayer, yoga, exercise, daydreaming, taking a nap in the afternoon, getting a massage, making love with someone you care deeply about, reading a good book, and laughing.

Get Involved in Group Activities

By supporting other people you are, in a sense, helping them to go beyond the limitations of fear. In this way you learn about the importance of support in the process of self-actualization.

See a Therapist, Take a Workshop, Get a Coach

Learn new life skills by participating in human-potential and personal-development seminars or workshops. (Note: human-potential and life-skill workshops should not be used in the place

> **Hornbeam:** This Bach Remedy helps overweight individuals deal with feelings of being tired, fatigued, or unable to face the day—feelings that create laziness, lack of energy, and more eating problems.
>
> **Impatiens:** This Bach Remedy relieves a sense of urgency or impatience with the slowness of others, impatience that may lead to frustration and may be acted out by excessive eating.
>
> **Larch:** This Bach Remedy boosts confidence and relieves the fear of failure that often causes people to slip from their weight-management programs.

of a skilled counselor or psychotherapist for the treatment of emotional or mental health problems.)

17 Ways to Test Yourself for Stress

1. Do you have a healthy breathing pattern, or are your breaths shallow and erratic? A healthy breathing pattern should be deep and regular.
2. Do you stop during the day to become aware of the way you are breathing?
3. Do you wear comfortable clothing that does not bind the waist, chest, or throat?
4. Do you sit in a relaxed, upright position with your spine relatively straight and your legs uncrossed? Or do you slouch and cross your legs?
5. When you are not feeling well, do you pay special attention to relaxing and breathing deeply? Or do you rush to get things done in spite of how you feel?
6. Do you practice daily meditation and visualization exercises for at least fifteen or twenty minutes each day?
7. Do you take twenty minutes daily to exercise?
8. Do you enjoy your job? If not, do you explore ways to make it more emotionally satisfying?

Mimulus: This Bach Remedy is especially valuable for those suffering from anorexia, bulimia, and other eating disorders because it relieves unreasonable phobias of known origin such as those related to spiders, the dark, public places, heights, being thin, feeling fat, etc.

Mustard: This Bach Remedy brings some clarity and relief from unexplained periods of emotional darkness or the blues, which may be caused by being overweight.

9. Do you make time every day to relax? Can you relax without feeling guilty about not working or not taking care of something important?
10. Do you take vacations? Do you think about work while you're on vacation?
11. Do you relax at meals and chew your food slowly, or do you eat in a hurry?
12. Are you at peace with yourself?
13. Are your personal relationships satisfying? Caring and loving relationships are essential for physical and emotional health.
14. Do you have friends with whom you can unburden yourself and from whom you can get good advice? Do you listen to the opinions of others, or do you think that you have all the answers?
15. Do you smoke or pick your nails? What habits do you have that are related to stress?
16. Do you communicate clearly, taking the time to say what you need to say slowly and articulately, or do you speak very quickly and rush through the ends of your sentences?
17. Do you enjoy the activities you use to manage your stress?

Thirty-four Ways to Reduce Stress

A lot of things are stressful simply because we don't allow ourselves enough time to get them done. Look for ways to take the

> **Oak:** This Bach Remedy helps a person to keep their mental, physical, and spiritual health at the forefront of their concerns on an ongoing basis. This is valuable for those individuals inclined to go on extreme low-calorie diets or nutritionally unbalanced weight-loss programs. Oak helps a person keep in mind the importance of going on a "balanced" weight-management program.
>
> **Olive:** This Bach Remedy is best used for mental and physical exhaustion and sapped vitality with no reserve. This may come on after an illness, a personal ordeal, or after a cycle of bingeing or yo-yo dieting.

hurry out of your everyday tasks and responsibilities.

1. Fill your life with a loving and supportive environment.
2. Get out of bed fifteen minutes earlier to avoid rushing around in the morning.
3. Prepare for the morning the evening before by setting out clothes, setting things up for breakfast, and preparing lunches.
4. Write things down; don't rely on your memory.
5. Take an extra minute to be sure that you understand anything that was said to you in order to save time and prevent aggravation.
6. Keep a duplicate car key in your wallet; bury a duplicate house key in your garden.
7. Practice "preventive maintenance" on your car, appliances, teeth, personal relationships, etc., so that they don't break down at the worst possible moment.
8. Eat healthful foods. Don't overeat. Always leave the table feeling a little hungry.
9. Whatever you want to do tomorrow, do it today; whatever you want to do today, do it now. Hard work is simply the accumulation of easy things you didn't do when you should have done them.

Pine: This Bach Remedy reduces the tendency to be hard on oneself to the extent of taking the blame for another's mistakes. The anxiety created by this kind of behavior can lead to overeating.

Red Chestnut: This Bach Remedy reduces worry over the hardships or misfortunes of loved ones. Worrying can lead to overeating.

10. Remember to pray or practice some form of spirituality.
11. Organize your home and work area so that everything has a place. You won't have to go through the stress of losing things.
12. Plan ahead. Don't let the gas tank get below one-quarter full; buy bus tokens and stamps before you need them.
13. Schedule a realistic day. Allow ample time between appointments. Make a "to do" list and cut it in half.
14. Relax your standards. The world will not end if the grass does not get mowed this weekend.
15. Engage in thirty minutes of brisk walking or some other aerobic exercise.
16. Make everyday purchases by cash or check.
17. Simplify.
18. Say, "No, thank you" to projects you don't have the time or energy to complete.
19. Always carry reading material to enjoy while waiting in lines or for appointments.
20. Remind yourself that Babe Ruth struck out 1,330 times.
21. For every one thing that goes wrong, remember that there are fifty to one hundred blessings. Count them.
22. Avoid doing anything that will cause you to tell a lie.
23. Put your brain in gear before opening your mouth. Before saying anything, ask yourself if what you are about to say is true, kind, and necessary. If it's not all three, D.S.A. (Don't Say Anything.)

Rock Rose: This Bach Remedy is helpful in reducing stress for for those who suffer from feelings of panic, terror, or nightmares. These people may turn to food to find a sense of safety as well as the peace, comfort, and emotional nourishment they are lacking. For these individuals food becomes a sort of security blanket.

Scleranthus: This Bach Remedy is valuable for those who have difficulty making decisions, including positive choices about eating and picking the best weight-reduction program for their individual needs.

Star of Bethlehem: This Bach Remedy helps to pacify the state of grief or trauma due to loss. Overweight people often turn to food during these times.

Sweet Chestnut: This Bach Remedy eases the feelings of despair that give you a sense that life is overwhelming or that you can't go on. Such feelings often lead to overeating.

Vervain: This Bach Remedy is useful for those who are argumentative and want to have the last word. These individuals often feel that no one is listening to them or were often told to keep quiet as children and are now compensating as adults. This "oral" frustration often results in overeating.

Vine: This Bach Remedy is good for individuals who are natural leaders or who feel the need to be in charge, possibly becoming dictatorial. Insecurity due to a weight problem can lead to this type of aggression.

Walnut: This Bach Remedy helps with sudden or extreme emotional transitions. These are often associated the types of hormonal changes that contribute to obesity.

24. If an unpleasant task faces you, do it early in the day and get it over with.
25. Write your thoughts and feelings in a journal. This can help you to clarify your ideas and put things in their proper perspective.
26. Get enough sleep. Use an alarm clock to remind you to go to bed, if necessary.
27. To relax instantly, breathe as if you were trying to inflate an imaginary balloon in your stomach. Inhale slowly to the count of ten, then exhale slowly to the count of ten. Repeat.
28. Don't put up with things that don't work right. Get them fixed or replace them.
29. Be kind to unkind people—they probably need it the most.
30. Unplug your phone or switch on your answering machine while you take a bath, have dinner, etc.
31. Make promises sparingly and keep them faithfully.
32. Buy clothes that are comfortable, easy and inexpensive to maintain, and easy to match with other clothes you already have.
33. Learn to enjoy quiet. Using the TV or radio for background "company" can be surprisingly stressful.
34. Forget about counting to ten. Count to one hundred before saying anything that could make matters worse.

The Most Popular Ways to Reduce Stress

1. Relaxation training
2. Visualization techniques
3. Exercise
4. Biofeedback training
5. Finding a quiet, secluded place (especially if you are often surrounded with noise, smoke, and crowds of people)
6. Calling a friend when confronted with the stress of loneliness, having a conversation with a colleague or

coworker to discuss an idea, or creating a solution to a problem you have been working on

7. Developing close and supportive personal relationships
8. Taking three-minute mini-breaks throughout your workday
9. Listening to quiet, soothing music through a portable cassette or CD player
10. Taking a short walk
11. Taking a fifteen minute nap
12. Doing deep breathing and relaxation exercises
13. Taking classes on time management
14. Learning self-massage or acupressure
15. Joining a support group or seeking professional guidance from a stress-management consultant
16. Getting a massage or acupressure session
17. Changing your attitude

Although there are many factors that determine a person's mental and emotional well-being, the one factor that is most within your control is the way you view life. If you have a poor attitude, everything will tend to seem negative and will be a source of fear. If you believe that life is to be lived fully and in celebration, then even the sad and hard times will not get you down for any longer than it takes for some genuine introspection.

18. Have an attitude that breeds joy and success

I am not just suggesting positive thinking. It's a wonderful concept, but it won't help you much when your world is collapsing around you. Maintaining an attitude that creates productive and effective choices, without or in spite of fear and anxiety, involves the ability to see all things as possible even if you do not intellectually understand how that is so. There is great power in being able to see that possibilities are available even when you are not feeling positive. The key to this is a willingness to conceive of yourself as deserving all of the best that life has to offer. Having this outlook about things is not something that comes automatically at first. It is something that develops over time and can be taught to you.

Water Violet: This Bach Remedy is helpful for those who prefer to bear emotional burdens on their own rather than seek the support of others. Many loners feel they must be self-reliant at all costs. This pattern can lead to the social isolation that results in overeating as compensation.

White Chestnut: This Bach Remedy is helpful to those with fast-moving, cluttered minds filled with the kind of constant chatter and diversions that makes concentration on healthy eating virtually impossible.

Dealing with Career-Based Stress

Actually, your goal is not to eliminate job stress, but to know when you've passed your stress maximum, then do something about it. If you're overstressed and you feel that your job is making so much of a demand on you that you can't handle it much longer, then it's time to develop a personal stress-management plan.

1. Find an off-the-job activity that gives you time off from stress. Relaxation and quiet time can work, as well as physical activity that allows you to release some of the tension you feel. Walking, jogging, tennis, and racquetball are all inexpensive activities that can give you a mini-vacation from your job. Once you find an activity that works well for you, make it a priority and commit yourself to one or two days a week at a specific time (or every day if you can manage it).

2. Identify personal habits that intensify stress. This can be hard is to do. Observe the ways in which you work. Are you a perfectionist, demanding too much of yourself and others? Do you rush through things that you might enjoy taking longer to do, whether it's business or pleasure? Do you constantly worry about "what if" scenarios? Be aware of your feelings and note when you feel most tense. Then

> **Wild Oat:** This Bach Remedy is good for those who are dissatisfied with their current situation in life or who feel as if they have not or cannot attain a goal they set for themselves. Being discouraged with life or oneself can create the frustration that leads to overeating.

think about the things you are presently doing or were doing just prior to these stressful feelings. Is the stress self-imposed? If so, how?

3. Once you've identified your stress-producing habits, write them down and keep the list handy so you can refer to it regularly. It will remind you to ease up and pace yourself.

4. Finally, learn how to handle job stress. Look at your job and list the people, tasks, and environmental factors that cause you stress. Next, identify ten stresses that occur repeatedly and rank them in order of highest (most frequent) to lowest. Then break down those stresses into three categories: those you can eliminate, those you can decrease or modify, and those you cannot control.

Focus on the least powerful stressor in the first category, determine how to eliminate it, and do so. Then congratulate yourself. Don't you feel better already? Continue through that category, then move on to the second category and see what progress you can make on the stresses there. Keep a log of how you handled each stressor so when others come along you'll know how to deal with them.

Conscious Eating

Once you develop the right attitude toward emotional well-being and stress, and have the key steps in place, it's time to create a system for choosing foods that will satisfy you. If you are going to be successful in losing weight, you will have to become conscious of what and how you eat while allowing your body to adapt to the process.

> **Wild Rose:** This Bach Remedy is great for those ready to begin a weight-management program. It is especially appropriate since a new program always involves a change and Wild Rose aids those with a desire to change their lives but have resigned themselves to their current positions.

Creating a successful program that satisfies your appetite and tastes while increasing your metabolism and reducing fat requires a number of specifics. Notice what time of day you enjoy eating most. Where do you like to eat? Do you enjoy cooking or would you prefer to eat out? Can you stop eating when you're full? Are you ever full?

What do you enjoy eating most? Are you attracted more to the taste of a food, the texture, or the aroma? What size portions do you prefer? Are you a gourmet eater or do you prefer simplicity?

Do you eat to live, or do you eat to feel love or to avoid feelings of sadness or loneliness? Do you throw discipline to the wind and eat high-fat junk foods at parties and during holiday celebrations? Do you have an extra glass of wine or an extra dessert during romantic dinners?

Can you be satisfied with eating a basic whole-food diet? Do you know the difference between whole foods and junk food? Do you define the quality of what you eat by the ingredients, the fat content, and how much the food has been processed?

Keys to Dieting Success

Consistency. Even if you keep strictly to the thirty-day program, your weight loss will not always be consistent. Many people lose as much as five to ten pounds of weight in the first week or two. This is simply "water weight," and not weight lost from fat burning. Over the days and weeks you will experience accelerated weight loss, which, at times, will plateau. The key to this program is to remain consistent.

Rock Water: This Bach Remedy is of value for those who like strict guidelines in everyday life and want to maintain an ideal, fulfill a goal (such as losing weight), or set an example.

Willow: This Bach Remedy reduces feelings of bitterness and resentment, often related to feeling as though one has been treated unfairly or dealt a bad hand in life. Such feelings can lead to overeating.

Keep it simple. Monitor your portions and chew your food well. Never eat less than twelve hundred calories a day unless you are fasting under the supervision of a physician or nutritional consultant. Be consistent in your meals and snacks as well as with the herbs and supplements.

Keep a food diary. If you think that you are keeping strictly to the program and are not losing weight, it may be time to take a closer look at you trouble spots. Keep a list of what, where, how, and when you eat. Do you eat more when you are angry, lonely, or sad? If so, you may need to find an outlet for this emotional stress that is not related to eating. This is where Bach Remedies come into play. At least one of the Bach Remedies will match your emotional needs, whatever your emotional issues concerning your weight. Review all of the remedies and see which one works best for you.

Chapter 7

Losing Weight with Living Juices

Many people find that drinking freshly extracted juices (also known as juice fasting because no solid food is used) and using herbal extracts and teas help them lose weight more effectively and keep it off. In juicing, almost 100 percent of the vital nutritive elements of fruits and vegetables are directly assimilated into the bloodstream without putting a strain on the digestive system.

Freshly pressed juices have been used in the last hundred years or so and as such are among the more recently discovered natural healing tools. They are a great source of easily absorbed nutrients and plant essences and have a powerful effect on the body's recuperative powers. One of the most important aspects of fresh juice therapy is the amount of enzymes the juices make available to the system. Plant food enzymes are the key to life and are extremely valuable on all levels of the healing and rehabilitation process.

According to N.W. Walker, a pioneer in the use of juice therapy in the United States, "The juices extracted from fresh raw vegetables and fruits are the means by which we can furnish all the cells and tissues of the body with the elements and the nutritional enzymes that they need, in the manner in which they can be most readily digested and assimilated" (Walker).

Digestive function, assimilation, and elimination are all assisted by the presence of enzymes. Enzymes help perform many biological processes without energy and without becoming

Spirulina: Spirulina is a type of micro algae. Micro algaes are aquatic plants that have no roots, leaves, seeds, or flowers. Many varieties are used in commercial weight-loss formulas because they are a rich source of nutrients that can easily be absorbed by the body. Because the minerals in algae are chelated (bonded) to amino acids, they have greater bio-availability and are easier for the body to fully use. Spirulina is a multi-cell, freshwater, blue/green algae, and is the micro algae most commonly found in herbal weight-loss formulas. Spirulina, which derives its name from the Latin word for "spiral," has been used as a food by tribes in Central America and Africa for centuries. It is now farmed and cultivated on a large scale in places such as California, Mexico, and Japan. Over the last several years, Spirulina has been used by many people as an effective aid to losing weight. Spirulina works in a number of ways:

1. Spirulina is an effective appetite suppressant. This may be because algae contains the amino acid phenylalanine, which is thought to act directly on the appetite center of the brain. Since Spirulina is a micro-nutrient (usually used in small amounts), it is taken as an ingredient in a commercial weight-loss formula or as a powder in smoothies and shakes.

2. On a pound for pound basis, Spirulina has a higher percentage of protein and B complex vitamins than any other vegetable or herbal source. As a comparison, note that Spirulina is 65 to 70 percent protein, containing all eight essential amino acids in perfect balance. By comparison, the protein content in eggs is 45 percent brewer's yeast, 40 percent soybeans, and 35 percent powdered and skim milk. To give you a sense of Spirulina protein content, beef, which is considered a high-protein food, contains only 22 percent protein.

3. Spirulina is a great source of vitamin E, has thirty-five times more beta-carotene than carrots, and more antioxi-

dant enzymes and pigments than found in any other food source. Most importantly for those on the herbal weight-loss program, Spirulina is high in the essential fatty acid Gamma-Linolenic Acid (GLA), containing more than evening primrose oil, one of the best sources. One tablespoon per day of Spirulina (ten grams) yields one hundred milligrams of GLA.

4. Chlorophyll is a valuable herbal/nutritional compound, and Spirulina is richer in chlorophyll than barley, wheat, or alfalfa extracts.

5. Spirulina contains substantial amounts of complete proteins, essential fatty acids, vitamins, and minerals while also being low in calories.

Since Spirulina is a food, it is quite safe and can be used like any other food. For dieting, however, best results come from taking this supplement either with breakfast or instead of breakfast, and then perhaps an hour before each of the other meals. Instructions come with the product, which also can be purchased in tablet form, but which usually is found as a powder. At the start, a single dose might be one half teaspoon in a glass of water, gradually increasing to a full teaspoon taken two or three times a day.

involved in the processes themselves. These enzymes serve as catalysts that help the body go on with its healing.

Six Tips for Weight Loss with Healing Juices

1. Use only freshly extracted juices. Canned and bottled juices are of limited or no value in a juice therapy program because they lack the living enzymes found in fresh extracted juice that are essential to restoring proper digestive function.

2. Drink juices immediately after extracting. Do not refrigerate or store for later use.

3. Use fresh fruits and vegetables. Green vegetables should

have full color. Avoid iceberg lettuce, blanched celery, etc.

4. Drink about a pint of juice daily if you are in a healthy state. If you are ill or on a purification program, it may be appropriate to drink sixteen-ounce portions of juice at least two to four times a day. Certain juices seem to have their greatest effect when combined with other juices. Among these are the juice of asparagus, beets and beet greens, dandelion, garlic, horseradish root, lemon, parsley, radish, spinach, and turnips.

5. Add a thermogenic herbal extract to each glass of juice that you drink.

6. Add a teaspoon of Spirulina micro algae to each glass of juice. Spirulina is available in most natural-food stores. It is a powerful balancer for those with impaired digestion. It is easily digested and it is a highly alkaline moderator that balances over-acidic body chemistry, a state that is common in those on high-fat diets.

Benefits of Freshly Extracted Juices

Fresh-pressed juices are rich in proteins, carbohydrates, enzymes, chlorophyll, aromatic oils, and other important healing and purifying components. They are also a great source of easily absorbed nutrients and plant essences, and have a powerful effect on the body's recuperative powers. The following list describes many of the purifying and healing elements to be found in fresh fruits and vegetables. Juice them and watch them help you lose weight.

Juicing Ingredients

Apples—A great source of pectin, potassium, and phosphorus. The potassium in apple juice helps lower blood pressure, and the fiber, especially pectin, helps eliminate the constipation that many obese people suffer.

Asparagus—Acts as an effective diuretic. Though this is not as important in the long run, it can be very motivating in the first week of your weight-loss program to lose excess water weight.

This juice is also very healing to the kidneys. It is especially valuable for breaking up the accumulation of oxalic acids throughout the body, thus reducing the potential for forming kidney stones.

Beets—Provide potassium, which helps lower blood pressure. Used by many healers as a blood-building tool.

Beet greens—Source of vitamin A, potassium, calcium, and iron.

Blueberry—An astringent, antiseptic, and blood purifier.

Brussels sprouts—Serves as a regenerator of pancreatic function and digestion. Especially useful in helping the body metabolize sugars more effectively. They are especially of value to those with hypoglycemia.

Cabbage—Source of sulfur, chlorine, and iodine. A great cleanser for the mucous membranes of the intestines and stomach.

Carrots—Provide beta-carotene, potassium, sodium, calcium, magnesium, and iron. Acts as a powerful aid to the maintenance of the bones and teeth and aids in liver and intestinal disorders.

Celery—Provides potassium, sodium, calcium, phosphorus, and magnesium.

Cucumber—Great source of chlorine, sulfur, and silicon. One of the most powerful diuretics among all juices. Helps in reducing water weight. Though this is not as important in the long run, it can be very motivating in the first week of your weight-loss program to lose excess water weight.

Dandelion—Source of potassium, calcium, sodium, magnesium, and iron. Counteracts hyperacidity.

Fennel—Powerful blood builder.

Garlic—Rich source of mustard oils and is an active cleanser of mucous from the sinus cavities and bronchial tubes. Garlic is best mixed in with other milder juices.

Grapefruit—Powerful source of vitamin C and potassium. Helpful in lowering blood pressure.

Kale—Many of the same properties as cabbage juice.

Leeks—Similar to garlic and onion juice in its effects, although leek juice is milder.

Lemon—Great source of vitamin C and bioflavonoids. Also acts as a potent cleanser of mucous.

Onion—Same healing properties as garlic juice but milder.

Parsnip (cultivated, not wild)—Provides chlorine, potassium, phosphorus, silicon, and sulfur.

Papaya—In its unripe state, papaya is high in the protein-digesting enzyme papain.

Parsley—Valuable source of vitamin C, vitamin A, calcium, magnesium, phosphorus, and potassium. Though this is not as important in the long run, it can be very motivating in the first week of your weight-loss program to lose excess water weight. Supports the adrenal and thyroid glands. Since it has a very intense taste it is best taken in two-ounce doses with other juices.

Potato—Provides chlorine, phosphorus, potassium, and sulfur. Stops muscle cramps.

Radish—Supplies potassium, sodium, iron, and magnesium, and acts as a blood builder.

Sorrel—Source of iron, magnesium, phosphorus, sulfur, and silicon. Promotes growth of nails and hair.

Tomato—Supplies sodium, calcium, potassium, and magnesium, and promotes healthy bones and gums.

Turnip—Source of perhaps the highest level of calcium of all juicing vegetables. Builds strong bones.

Eliminating Yo-Yo Dieting with Juices and Herbal Extracts

Many people bounce from diet to diet, struggling to lose unwanted weight. If you apply this program wisely you will be able to lose inches from your waistline through a combination of liquid herbal extracts and juicing. It is an easy three-step program that you will find can naturally control your appetite while feeding your sweet tooth in a totally healthy way.

Begin each morning by having a sixteen-ounce glass of homemade juice. Add the liquid extracts of two important herbs, Gymnema sylvestre and Garcinia cambogia, to your daily juice.

> **Gymnema sylvestre:** This herb, also know as gurmar, has been used in Ayurvedic for over two thousand years to control problems in carbohydrate metabolism, particularly concerning obesity and diabetes. Recent studies have confirmed that it reduces blood glucose levels, in part by preventing the intestine from absorbing sugar molecules. In addition, research has shown that Gymnema sylvestre extracts increase liver and pancreatic function. Dysfunction and weakness in these organs have been shown to be a factor in obesity.
>
> Another valuable aspect of this herb is that it appears to reduce cravings for sweet foods through its influence on the taste receptors. It also aids in the uptake of oxygen into the cells. Gymnema sylvestre functions as an insulin potentiator and appears to normalize blood lipid levels and lower insulin requirements.

These herbs are available in combination from most health-food stores. Use twenty drops Gymnema sylvestre/Garcinia cambogia liquid extract.

Homemade Mixed Vegetable Juice
Ingredients:
> 2 cups canned tomatoes
> ½ to ¾ cup celery pieces or tops
> 1 piece of sweet red or green pepper
> 1 wedge of Red leaf, Romaine, or Boston lettuce
> ½ cup carrot pieces
> 1 piece of cabbage
> 1 large sprig of parsley
> 1 piece of sweet onion or onion top
> 1 tsp. of vegetable seasoning (such as Vegebase Brand,
>   available in your health-food store)
> 20 drops Gymnema sylvestre/Garcinia cambogia liquid extract

Preparation Instructions:
Blend the mixture until it's thick and smooth. Add ice cubes at the

> **Garcinia cambogia:** This herb is made from a dried jungle berry native to India. This is among the most effective and balanced of the herbs that promote weight loss. It is rich in hydroxycitric acid (also called hydrocitrate or HCA). The HCA is extracted from the dried rind of the fruit. It has been shown to curb the appetite, increase the burning of calories, reduce fat production and storage, reduce cholesterol synthesis, inhibit the conversion of carbohydrates (sugars) into fat, and improve the rate of fat burning in cells by inhibiting an enzyme that blocks fat from being burned (malonyl CoA). In addition, it not only can curb your appetite, but also aids digestion and reduces cravings for sweets.
>
> The prevailing theory is that it prevents carbohydrates from converting to fat in the body. Instead, they convert to glycogen, a more easily usable form of energy. HCA also helps reduce the formation of a key enzyme, the lack of which reduces the production of undesirable low-density lipoprotein and triglycerides. Preliminary studies suggest that the effectiveness of HCA is increased when it is used in conjunction with niacin-bound chromium (chromium polynicotinate).

end to cool it and make it smoother. You can add some lime juice or cayenne to zest it up. Generally, the taste will be similar to the canned V-8 juice you can buy.

Throughout the day, alternate fresh fruit salads with vegetable juices. You will not only lose your excess weight, but you will gain an increased youthfulness, health, and vibrancy.

More Purifying Than a Fast

Health spas have become more popular than ever, and today almost all health spas and clinics employ juice-fasting. Most of the leading authorities on health and nutrition agree that fasting on fresh, raw fruit and vegetable juices, with the addition of vegetable broth and herb teas, will result in faster recovery from disease and a more effective cleansing of toxic wastes than a water fast. You, too, can bring the benefits of an expensive spa into your home by introducing juices into your daily regime.

Using this juice purification program, you will discover a renewed energy and vitality, which will seem to carve years off of your biological age as well as excess weight off of your body. The juice purification program is an easy and efficient way to not only improve your skin tone but also to put a spring in your step and a new lightness in your life. Juicing is a great way to lose weight while cleansing your bloodstream and vital organs.

Seven Days of Purification with Juices and Thermogenic Herbs

Here is my favorite juice-herb combination program. Try it for a day or two and when you find how much it does for you, you can continue with it for up to seven days.

Upon Rising:

Drink one eight-ounce glass of freshly squeezed citrus juice (orange or grapefruit) or one half of a lemon, squeezed into a glass of distilled water. This is rich in vitamin C, which helps to strengthen your blood vessels.

Mid-Morning:

Have one cup of Purification Tea* (see recipe in appendix) with a small amount of honey if desired. This will flush out toxins from your internal organs.

Noon:

Drink one large glass of freshly extracted Basic Cleansing Juice, consisting of carrots, celery, and parsley (see recipe in appendix). This drink is rich in minerals and beta-carotene and will strengthen the immune system.**

Evening:

Have a bowl of warm potassium broth or a glass of fresh vegetable juice. ***This will help replenish the body's minerals.

Before Retiring:

Again, enjoy a cup of Purification Tea with a small amount of honey if desired.

*If you wish, Purification Tea can be alternated with other milder teas, such as peppermint, chamomile, or rose hips. All three of these herbs have healing properties. Chamomile is a relaxant and is superb for the digestive system. It makes a good nighttime tea. Rose hip has a high vitamin C content, which is helpful for detoxification during fasting. Peppermint is an excellent overall restorative herb.

**The ideal combination is five parts carrot, two parts celery, and one-half part parsley. (Parsley should be taken in small quantities due to its high iron content.) Carrot-apple is another popular mixture. Combine in any way you like. These formulas help to flush out the kidneys.

***If you want to expand beyond just juicing, I recommend vegetable broth, which can be made by gathering various vegetables (i.e., potatoes, carrots, broccoli, string beans, cauliflower, celery, turnips, cabbage, onions, sea vegetables, etc.), and cooking them in distilled water in a large pot for about thirty minutes (low flame), then straining. This type of broth is both cleansing and building.

When you're thirsty, drink distilled water with fresh lemon juice added to taste. Your total juice and broth intake for the day should be between one and one and one-half quarts.

Mild exercise during the day will highly benefit you during your juice-fast. Walking, or jogging if you are used to it, are excellent forms of exercise.

Juice Therapy

Unless you are on a supervised juice therapy herbal program, you should avoid most fruit juices while you are following a weight-loss program. Many dieters drink large quantities of juices because they consider them to be low in calories. However, many fruit juices are high in calories and do not provide the benefits of fiber.

Here is one juice formula that you will find helpful, however. Add one teaspoon of bee pollen to a sixteen-ounce mixture of carrot, beet, and apple juice. This formula will help support your glandular function.

Your Home Guide to Preparing Fresh Juices and Blended Drinks

Some individuals like the idea of juicing, but either do not own a juicer or do not want to lose the fiber that a juicer removes. For these individuals I recommend blended drinks. Blended drinks are rich in fiber, which make them more filling than juice alone. Either is acceptable and can be used as a meal replacement of one meal a day if you are not fasting.

Preparing Fruits and Vegetables for the Blender

Fruits and vegetables only need washing and cutting up. If organically grown, no peeling is necessary; however, if bought in a regular market, then washing and peeling is recommended. Celery will blend smoothly, including strings. If you are using hot broth, any vegetable or cooked beans or grains can be added.

To get the smoothest consistency in your blended drink:

1. Start the blender at about one-quarter to one-third full of liquid.
2. Cut the vegetables and fruits into chunks and add them slowly while the blender is on. (This might save you getting a chunk of something hard like a carrot stuck in the blades.)
3. Keep the mixture thick, adding more liquid as it thickens.
4. To increase the smooth consistency, you can add a banana or ice cubes or both. Ice also cools the drink and makes it more appetizing.
5. Pour into a serving pitcher and thin with juice to taste.

Get the Most Out of Your Blended Drinks

Add any of the following for a refreshing, nutrition-rich, body-purifying beverage.

- Fresh vegetables of any kind, (carrots, celery, beets, cabbage, asparagus, etc.)
- Fresh fruits of any kind (bananas, apples, oranges, peaches, grapes, etc.)
- Rice beverage or soy milk

- A teaspoon of flaxseed
- Twenty drops Gymnema sylvestre/Garcinia cambogia liquid extract

Low-Fat, Low-Calorie Breakfast Elixirs

Start with the liquid you want to use. Some of the most popular are unsweetened apple juice, V-8 bottled juice (only if you cannot make fresh juice), tomato juice, and unsweetened papaya concentrate (from a health-food store).

You can also make your own nut and seed milks by blending them with distilled water.

1. Fill the blender about one-quarter full of juice or liquid.
2. Place a layer of something soft like cabbage pieces in the blender.
3. Add pieces of carrot, beet, and apple, and blend. To get it as smooth as possible, keep it thick.
4. When everything you want to add seems to be as smooth as possible, add a banana, flaxseed, some ice cubes, and also some pineapple juice if it's getting too thick.

My Favorite Blended Drink Recipes
Pineapple/Vegetable Cocktail
Ingredients:

8 oz. pineapple juice
1 large beet or 2 or 3 smaller ones, cut up
1 large carrot or several smaller ones, cut up
1 or 2 Jerusalem artichokes (sun chokes), pieces of celery, parsley, etc.
1 banana and ice cubes
20 drops Gymnema sylvestre/Garcinia cambogia liquid extract

Preparation Instructions:

Add liquid until the blender is one-fourth full and keep adding ingredients until the mixture is thick.

Sparkling Orange Cranberry Punch
Ingredients:
½ cup either fresh or frozen raw cranberries
½ cup orange juice
¼ cup honey
1 cup sodium free sparkling water
1 apple
20 drops Gymnema sylvestre/Garcinia cambogia liquid extract

Preparation Instructions:
Blend the mixture until it is thick and smooth. Blend and strain the mixture through a wire strainer, shaking and stirring the mixture to keep it straining. Don't rub it through the strainer too hard in order to keep the punch clearer.

Add enough water to make about a quart of punch. This will still be strong enough so you will be able to add ice to the punch bowl. Repeat and make as many batches as you need for your punch bowl.

You can serve the cranberries left in the strainer as a relish either alone or mixed with nuts, grapes, pineapple, etc.

Alternate ingredients for a high-protein fruit smoothie:

Fresh peach—Use one-fourth cup honey, one-half teaspoon almond flavoring, and four medium peaches.

Fresh apricot—Same as peach, using seven unpeeled, halved apricots.

Red fruits—Cranberry, strawberry, raspberry. Use one cup unsweetened fruit plus five tablespoons honey.

Dark fruits, blueberries, etc.—Use one and one-half cups of fresh fruit and five tablespoons of honey. Use vanilla flavoring to taste.

Yellow or orange colored fruits—Use one cup of fresh fruit and almond flavoring, alone or with vanilla plus five tablespoons honey.

Papaya juice—Use one cup in place of fruit plus five tablespoons honey. You can adjust the amount of honey you add to suite your taste.

Green Pineapple Splash
Ingredients:
> 2 Tbsp. raw, unsalted sunflower seeds
> 1 tsp. Spirulina
> 1 tsp. Flaxseed
> ¼ cup pineapple juice
> 1 cup plain rice or soy beverage
> 20 drops Gymnema sylvestre/Garcinia cambogia
>   liquid extract
> 6 ice cubes

Preparation Instructions:
Mix all of the above ingredients in a blender for one minute or until smooth.

Tropical Quencher
Ingredients:
> ¼ cup pineapple chunks
> ¼ cup mango chunks
> ½ banana (sliced)
> 1 cup low-fat milk
> 20 drops Gymnema sylvestre/Garcinia cambogia
>   liquid extract
> 6 ice cubes

Preparation Instructions:
Mix all of the above ingredients in a blender for one minute or until frothy.

Banana Soymilk Smoothie
Ingredients:
> ¼ tsp. cinnamon powder
> 1 cup plain soy beverage
> ¼ cup banana pieces
> 20 drops Gymnema sylvestre/Garcinia cambogia
>   liquid extract

Preparation Instructions:
Mix apple pieces well; add cinnamon; place in a freezable dish and allow to become firm. When all components are ready, mix well and enjoy.

This recipe should be sweet enough with the banana, but you can add some easily digestible sweeteners that are available at your local natural-food store. Add barley malt syrup, rice syrup, or a few drops of Stevia.

CarbBerry Heaven
Ingredients:
> 4-5 raspberries (fresh or unsweetened frozen)
> 2 strawberries (fresh or unsweetened frozen)
> 3 Tbsp. blueberries (fresh or unsweetened frozen)
> 1 cup rice beverage
> 20 drops Gymnema sylvestre/Garcinia cambogia
>   liquid extract
> 6 ice cubes

Preparation Instructions:
Mix all of the above ingredients in a blender for one minute or until smooth.

Balanced Carbo-Protein Herbal Smoothie
Ingredients:
> 2 cups of unsweetened frozen or fresh berries (1 banana)
> 1 cake of soft silken tofu
> 1 tsp. of sugar-free vanilla extract
> 1 tsp. flaxseed
> 20 drops Gymnema sylvestre/Garcinia cambogia
>   liquid extract

Preparation Instructions:
Blend well and add:
> 1 cup ice cubes or until thick.

Citrus Lymphatic Flush
Ingredients:
> *4 large grapefruits*
> *3 medium lemons*
> *3 quarts distilled water*

This formula is used to re-alkanalize the body and cleanse the lymphatic system. It is best used over a two to three day period as part of a fast. Approximately six ounces is taken every thirty minutes until the entire mixture has been taken. At the end of the day take a glass of celery/carrot combination.

Herbal Liver Flush

As your body is purifying, the liver plays an important role in the process. It is for this reason that the liver must be specifically cleansed as well. One of the most effective ways for doing this is the Liver Flush. This is based on a classic formula developed by Dr. Randolph Stone, the founder of Polarity Therapy. Many herbalists use it. Every morning, prepare a liver-cleansing tea.

Ingredients:
> *l tsp. olive oil*
> *½ tsp. fresh chopped or grated ginger*
> *l tsp. fenugreek (a seed found in health-food stores)*
> *The juice of one whole lemon*
> *A pinch of capsicum (cayenne pepper)*

Preparation Instructions:

Take one cup of boiled, distilled water, letting it cool for one or two minutes. Add these ingredients (add the olive oil when you are ready to drink it). Strain the mixture and drink the remaining liquid. If you wish, you can throw the entire mixture in a blender and drink the liquefied ingredients. Though some people may find the taste unusual, it is a powerful cleanser for the liver, the digestive tract, and the intestines.

Losing Weight through the Influence of Enzymes

One of the most important aspects of fresh-juice therapy as a system for weight loss is the amount of enzymes that it makes available to the system. Plant-food enzymes are extremely valuable on all levels of the weight-management process. When the level of nutrition that the body is able to absorb is increased, you feel satisfied from your food intake without needing to eat large amounts of calories. Following are my favorite enzyme-rich formulas. When drinking them or any of the morning shakes or elixirs, take Garcinia cambogia capsules or extract, since this herb cannot only curb your appetite but also aids digestion and reduces cravings for sweets. Combine the juices in the following recipes.

Recipe No. 1

> 4 oz. carrot
> 6 oz. cucumber
> 2 oz. beet
> 4 oz. apple
> 20 drops Gymnema sylvestre/Garcinia cambogia
>   liquid extract

Use this recipe during the first two weeks of your weight-management program.

Warning: do not use if you have low blood sugar or diabetes.

Recipe No. 2

> 5 oz. carrot
> 8 oz. celery
> 3 oz. parsley
> 20 drops Gymnema sylvestre/Garcinia cambogia
>   liquid extract

This is recommended for weak digestion.

Use this recipe during the first two weeks of your weight-management program.

Warning: do not use if you have low blood sugar or diabetes.

Recipe No. 3

> 4 oz. carrot
> 4 oz. apple
> 2 oz. beet
> 6 oz. cucumber
> 20 drops Gymnema sylvestre/Garcinia cambogia
>   liquid extract

Use this recipe during the first two weeks of your weight-management program.

Warning: do not use if you have low blood sugar or diabetes.

Recipe No. 4

> 10 oz. cucumber
> 4 oz. carrot
> 2 oz. raw potato
> 20 drops Gymnema sylvestre/Garcinia cambogia liquid extract

Recipe No. 5

> 2 oz. pear
> 2 oz. kale
> 2 oz. carrot
> 5 oz. asparagus
> 5 oz. cucumber
> 20 drops Gymnema sylvestre/Garcinia cambogia liquid extract

Recipe No. 6

> 7 oz. carrot
> 6 oz. cucumber
> 2 oz. parsley
> 20 drops Gymnema sylvestre/Garcinia cambogia liquid extract

Recipe No. 7

    4 oz. carrot

    6 oz. cucumber

    2 oz. beet

    3 oz. parsley

    20 drops Gymnema sylvestre/Garcinia cambogia liquid extract

Recipe No. 8

    6 oz. cabbage

    6 oz. cucumber

    4 oz. grapefruit

    20 drops Gymnema sylvestre/Garcinia cambogia liquid extract

Warning: do not use if you suffer from colitis.

Recipe No. 9

    10 oz. carrot

    3 oz. celery

    3 oz. cabbage

    20 drops Gymnema sylvestre/Garcinia cambogia liquid extract

Recipe No. 10

    14 oz. carrot

    lemon juice (one-half of a lemon squeezed)

    horseradish root (grate ½ tsp. of this root into the carrot juice)

Recipe No. 11

    4 oz. apple

    2 oz. beet

    4 oz. carrot

    4 oz. celery

    2 oz. spinach

    20 drops Gymnema sylvestre/Garcinia cambogia liquid extract

Warning: those who suffer from kidney stones should remove the spinach from this juice combination.

Recipe No. 12
    6 oz. carrot
    6 oz. celery
    2 oz. beet and beet tops
    2 oz. alfalfa sprouts
    20 drops Gymnema sylvestre/Garcinia cambogia liquid extract

Recipe No. 13
    7 oz. carrot
    5 oz. green pepper
    20 drops Gymnema sylvestre/Garcinia cambogia liquid extract

Recipe No. 14
    5 oz. Brussels sprouts
    2 oz. carrot
    5 oz. string beans
    2 oz. escarole lettuce
    20 drops Gymnema sylvestre/Garcinia cambogia liquid extract

Recipe No. 15
    6 oz. carrot
    3 oz. celery
    7 oz. escarole lettuce
    20 drops Gymnema sylvestre/Garcinia cambogia liquid extract

Recipe No. 16
    10 oz. carrot
    3 oz. dandelion
    3 oz. turnip leaves
    20 drops Gymnema sylvestre/Garcinia cambogia liquid extract

Recipe No. 17

    6 oz. carrot

    3 oz. spinach

    3 oz. turnip leaves

    4 oz. watercress lettuce

    20 drops Gymnema sylvestre/Garcinia cambogia liquid extract

Recipe No. 18

    6 oz. carrot

    4 oz. celery

    3 oz. parsley

    3 oz. spinach

    20 drops Gymnema sylvestre/Garcinia cambogia liquid extract

Recipe No. 19

    3 oz. carrot

    6 oz. cucumber

    4 oz. celery

    1 oz. beets

    20 drops Gymnema sylvestre/Garcinia cambogia liquid extract

Recipe No. 20

    8 oz. carrot

    2 oz. cucumber

    6 oz. celery

    20 drops Gymnema sylvestre/Garcinia cambogia liquid extract

Recipe No. 21

    8 oz. carrot

    8 oz. celery

    20 drops Gymnema sylvestre/Garcinia cambogia liquid extract

Recipe No. 22
    8 oz. beet
    7 oz. romaine lettuce
    l oz. dandelion
    20 drops Gymnema sylvestre/Garcinia cambogia liquid extract

In addition to juice formula recommendations, Purification Tea can be taken throughout the day.

Chapter 8

Thinning with Culinary Herbs and Spices

Culinary herbs and spices help people lose weight and stay thin by adding low-calorie texture, aromas, and flavors to food that would ordinarily be higher in fat.

Many people become confused by the difference between an herb and a spice. The English, whose large shipping fleets helped expand the use of different herbs and spices throughout the world, generally referred to spices when describing tropical plants with aromatic fruits or barks, and herbs when discussing plants of temperate climates featuring aromatic leaves. This distinction is no longer in practice. It might be said that, generally speaking, herbs are the leaves of fresh or dried plants, while spices are the aromatic parts of the plant—usually dried buds, fruits, berries, roots, or bark. In Asia this distinction is not so clear. Many sea plants, known in the West as sea vegetables or seaweed, are used as herbs and spices as well.

Traditionally, apart from the measures necessary for drying and packaging, commercially packaged spices should not be technically modified or mixed with any other components unless special names are applied to these mixtures, such as curry powder, soy sauce, or mixed pizza seasoning. In recent years there has been some controversy over the use of genetic engineering and the genetic modification of herbs and spices. For this reason it is best to buy herbs and spices that are labeled organically grown.

> **Seaweed:** Seaweeds (sea vegetables) are rich in polysaccharides, which form mucilage in contact with water; this mucilage distends the stomach without being absorbed. This quality makes it a wonderful appetite suppressant by giving a person a sense of fullness. It also has a slight laxative effect, which makes it useful in body detoxification. Seaweeds are also useful for general fatigue due to its stimulating action on the general metabolism, and for certain hormonal deficiencies, when an iodine supplement is necessary to treat obesity.

Among the earliest of herbal cookbooks was one written in the first century, attributed to the Roman epicurean Apicus. This book describes the use of herb combinations as flavor enhancers.

Looking through the recipe books and cookbooks of many different cultures, I have found that there are at most forty different spice plants used globally. There certainly are many more used locally in the regions of their natural origin.

Many of these can be found in ethnic restaurants or by immigrants who have maintained their cooking and herbal healing traditions. Sadly, many spices that enjoyed great popularity over the centuries have become obsolete and are now not even known to people in the West—especially since other cheaper spices with similar qualities became available.

What Makes a Spice a Spice?

I have included fifty-two different herb and spice plants in this chapter. Each plant has a specific taste, texture, and/or aromatic quality that makes it recognizable to your senses. These unique qualities come from the constituents in the plant. The constituents that are responsible for the spicy properties of plants are generally secondary metabolism products, that is, they are not vital for the plant. Although a large number of classes of plant constituents exist, most plants contain only a few of them. Only a small fraction of the many biochemicals found in plants are essential for spices. In large amounts, some of these biochemicals may even be toxic, but in very small amounts they are what make these spices rich in flavor and aroma.

As mentioned earlier, spices add texture, aroma, and flavor to food. These qualities come from biochemicals in the herbs including the following:

- *Alkaloids*—These are an important class of biochemicals that contain several well-known poisons and medicines. The pungent taste of chilies and black pepper are derived from biochemicals closely related to alkaloids. Glycosides are contained in mustard oil, white mustard seeds, and in horseradish.

- *Anethole, methylchavicol,* and *anisaldehyde*—The licorice flavor of *anise* is derived from a combination of three biochemical agents. These are anethole, methylchavicol, and anisaldehyde. Methylchavicol is related to chavicol, one of the agents that gives black pepper its sharp taste. Anisaldehyde has a faint vanilla-like flavor, which, when combined with the other agents, gives anise its flavor.

- *Carotenoides*—These are found in all plants. Several vegetables and fruits owe their orange color to them including carrots, cantaloupes, saffron, and paprika.

- *Eugenol*—This is found in cloves.

- *Fruit acids*—Can include many different biochemicals including citric acid, tartric, and malic acid. All these acids exhibit the sour taste we associate with lemon, orange, pomegranate, or mango.

- *Lipids*—These are commonly known as oils if liquid and fats if solid. Lipids occur in the plant kingdom primarily in seeds. In addition to contributing flavors of their own, oils absorb aroma compounds more easily than in water, so small amounts of vegetable oil will tend to improve the taste of every dish, since they extract the aroma from the spice pieces.

- *Monoterpenes*—These are formed in all plant families, but are most common and highly concentrated in the mint

family (Lamiaceae) and the parsley family (Apiaceae), both
of which contain a large number of culinary spice plants.

- *Phenylpropanoids*—These are found in cinnamon.
- *Safrol*—This can be toxic in high levels and is found in
  sassafras and nutmeg.
- *Sesquiterpenes*—These are of some importance for the
  fragrance of cinnamon and conifers (juniper), and take an
  important part in the aroma of ginger and other plants of
  the ginger family (Zingiberaceae), like turmeric and
  galangale.
- *Sulphur compounds*—These release the strong odor
  prominent in the onion family.
- *Tannines*—These are found in rosemary and sumac.
- *Terpenes*—This is the most important category of aroma
  compounds that include the phenol thymol, which is
  responsible for the aroma of thyme and ajwain.
- *Vanillin*—This is found in vanilla beans.

How to Best Use Spices

If you have the time and the inclination, it is almost always best to
use whole spices; grinding may be performed with a coffee mill
(don't use it for coffee anymore!).

Ground spices generally produce a fine powder that tends to
release the aromatic oils quickly. Ground spices are more susceptible to degradation during storage, causing loss of aroma and
some taste. It is best to store ground spices in a cool, dry, and dark
environment.

Some spices such as ginger and cinnamon are, because of their
firmer texture, difficult to grind at home. In such a case, it is probably best to buy these spices in powder form, but in small
amounts.

Some spices are not easy to obtain in their whole form.
Examples are paprika and cayenne pepper. Both of these are generally sold in powdered form. Whenever you buy herbs in powdered form, try to purchase them organically grown and in small

quantities, and use them as soon as possible. This also applies to most spice mixtures like curry and chili powder.

Culinary Herbs

Agar-Agar (Gelidium amansii): Derived from seaweed, this clear vegetable substance looks like transparent straw and is often used to replaces animal gelatin in jams and jellies and other desserts for vegetarians and those who prefer a natural food program. When I cook with agar-agar, I add one tablespoon for every cup of boiling water. Agar-agar doesn't look or taste like what you would expect a sea herb to look and taste like. But once you boil it in fruit juice or add it to blended bananas with a teaspoon of peanut butter, it makes a great sugar-free dessert. And it is a great intestinal cleanser as well.

Allspice (Pimenta dioica, Pimenta officinalis): Allspice is the fruit of an evergreen tree native to the West Indies and parts of Central and South America. Its name derives from the fact that it tastes like a combination of cloves, cinnamon, juniper berries, and other spices. These dried, whole berries may be used in pickling liquids or in spicing drinks. I use ground allspice in sauces, soups and dips, cakes, pies, and other desserts. When I'm experimenting, I use allspice combined with powdered nutmeg or cinnamon. Allspice is sometimes used as a replacement in recipes for ground cloves or ground cinnamon.

Anise Seed (Pimpinella anisum): A member of the carrot family and Native to Egypt and western Asia, anise tastes like licorice and is used in many ethnic types of cooking, especially breads, candy, stewed fruits, fruit pies, vegetable stews, hot or cold spiced beverages, cheese, salad dressings, and appetizers. Many people have been known to make anise seed into a soothing tea before going to bed since it is both a sleep aid and soothing for the digestive tract.

Arrowroot (Maranta arundinacea): Arrowroot is a starch made from the rhizomes of a plant native to the West Indies. This herb has very little flavor of its own, but it can influence the texture of any dish. It is principally used as a thickening agent in sauces, baked goods, gravy, soups, stews, and desserts, and as a healthy replacement for refined cornstarch. Because arrowroot powder cooks at a low temperature, it is ideal for use in sauces, which might otherwise burn easily. Arrowroot makes a clear sauce as opposed to cornstarch and flour, which produce a white, cloudy sauce. Arrowroot is used in the same measurement as cornstarch, is easy to digest, and has a pleasant almost neutral taste. It is useful for those individuals who have an allergic sensitivity to corn.

Basil (Ocimum basilicum): Commonly referred to as "sweet basil" or "garden basil," this spice is a member of the mint family. Native to Africa, India, and Asia, this spice adds a refreshingly warm flavor to foods such as classic Italian dishes including pesto dishes, pizza, and many tomato dishes. Greek and Italian cuisine emphasize basil, thyme, sage, and oregano.

Bay Leaves (Laurus nobilis): Also known as "sweet bay" or "noble laurel," these leaves have a tangy taste that adds flavor to vegetable soups, stews, sauces, tomato soup, and marinades for tofu, tempeh, and seitan (wheat gluten). Bay leaves are also used in French or herb salad dressings. I usually place the bay leaves in a small cheese cloth packet that I make up and add when I'm preparing barbecue or spaghetti sauce, since the edges of the whole herb can be pointy and sharp.

Caraway Seed (Carum carvi): This popular culinary spice, noted for its fragrant, almost licoricy, taste, is native to Asia and is a member of the carrot and parsley family. Interestingly, the caraway seed is actually the fruit of the plant, which, when ripe and dried, looks like a seed. Commonly used in baking, cooking, and salads, it is caraway seeds that we see in most rye bread. Caraway seeds can also be added to sauerkraut, potatoes, stews, cauliflower, and cottage cheese. Caraway seeds are often added to many different herbal and pekoe tea blends to add a sweet taste without sugar.

In many cultures, caraway is eaten at the end of the meal or taken as a tea since it is mildly carminative; that is, a cup of caraway tea can be used to expel unwanted gas from the body and settle upset stomachs.

Cardamom (Elettaria cardamomum): Native to India though widely cultivated elsewhere, especially the Middle East and Iran, the cardamom "seed" is actually the fruit of the plant. It is widely used as a flavoring in Asia in curry powders, baked goods, and as a flavorful addition to many of my favorite cooked dishes, including pies and vegetables. On cold winter nights, I make a beverage of a grain-based coffee substitute (Postum, Cafex, and Bambu are variations of this beverage) with rice or soy milk and add cardamom. It's my homemade version of an Indian tea called chai.

Cassia (Cinamomum cassia): Native to China, cassia is an evergreen member of the laurel family. Among herbalists, the bark and buds—cassia buds are the dried fruit of the cassia tree—are known as Chinese cinnamon or "false cinnamon" since it is a relative of "true" cinnamon, with which it is commonly mixed and sold in its ground form. The bark is sometimes marketed as cinnamon sticks in a rolled, scroll-like shape. In taste, cassia is stronger and more bitter than cinnamon. Cassia is a luscious tasting spice with a quality that reminds one of a combination of both cloves and cinnamon. It is a great addition to many desserts. Oil of cinnamon, which is found in both the bark and the bud, helps to break up intestinal gas.

Cayenne Pepper (Capsicum frutescens): Native to tropical America, cayenne is a perennial in the wild. The name of this spice comes from the Greek word *kapto*, which means "I bite," because of its zesty taste. Often called African Pepper, the fruit of the cayenne plant is used as a penetrating spice that adds heat and a firey accent to any dish and can be used in appetizers, soups, entrees, and desserts. It provides a great source of vitamin C and helps increase circulation.

Celery Seeds (Apium graviolens): Celery seeds are the dried fruit of a biennial plant native to Europe, Africa, and the Americas. The seeds are quite tiny and give a subtle seasoning to soups, salads, and tempeh and tofu dishes. I use ground celery seeds to flavor salads that call for celery. Celery has a slight salti-ness to it and, when combined with onion and garlic, can reduce the need to add salt to foods. An extract of celery seeds can be mixed with sparkling water and maple syrup or honey to create a Celery Soda.

Chervil (Anthriscus cerefolium): Also known as French pars-ley and as "gourmet's parsley," the name Chervil comes from the Greek word meaning "to rejoice," apparently referring also to the plant's fragrance.

It is an annual plant that is a member of the carrot family and is cultivated in many parts of the world as a kitchen spice. It is particularly popular with chefs trained in Western Europe. Chervil has the rich fragrance of common parsley that most cooks are familiar with.

Chia Seeds: Deriving from the Mexican sage plant, these seeds are used in bread and muffins and also in making teas. Many herbalists use them to increase energy in people who suffer from fatigue. I add it into blended smoothies with chlorella or some other micro algae, banana, or bee pollen. This chia seed is the same seed that is sold with those funny little ceramic faces that are advertised on television that you water and watch grow.

Chili Powder: This is a spice mixture created in the American Southwest in the nineteenth century consisting primarily of cayenne pepper. Rich in capsaicin, which promotes perspiration, cayenne is usually mixed with other components (cayenne, garlic powder, cumin, salt, and oregano) to form chili powder, a good source of betacarotene. Chilies have strong thermogenic properties and are thus a spice of choice for those on weight-loss programs.

Chili Peppers: These may produce an extremely hot flavor and are often added to soups and sauces. They are an essential season-ing in many Tex-Mex, Mexican-American, Indian, Mexican, and Middle Eastern dishes. I think people who like very hot chilies are those who in another time and place would have been the types to live dangerously. With chili pepper, you get to feel like you're liv-ing dangerously without any of the risk.

Chives (Allium schoenoprasum): Chives are a delicate-tasting member of the onion family. Native to Northern Europe and Asia, they are cultivated around the world for their pleasantly flavored leaves. Chives promote digestion and contain significant amounts of iron. The oils in chives have been found to lower blood levels of Low-Density Lipoproteins (LDL). Chives, in their dehydrated form, can be used liberally in many kinds of cooking, especially in dips, tofu cream cheese, and with stir-fried vegetables, baked potatoes, tofu dishes, gravies, and vegetables.

Cilantro (Coriandum sativum): *Cilantro* is the Spanish name applied to young, flat leaves of the spice known as coriander. Also known as Chinese parsley, it exhibits a taste similar to a blend of lime and parsley. Cilantro is often used in Asian and Mexican recipes, especially combined with various chili peppers and, more recently, epazot leaves to give a kick to refried beans.

Cinnamon (Cinnamomum zeylanicum): Native to Sri Lanka, this ancient spice is still one of the most common seasonings used today. Ground cinnamon is used as a spicy sweetener in baking and cooking, as well as in beverages. I use it in the preparation of rice pudding, hot spiced drinks, and fruit punches.

Cloves (Caryophyllus armoaticus, Syzygium aromaticum): A member of the myrtle family, Cloves are the dried flower buds of an evergreen tree native to Indonesia and the Philippines. Cloves were introduced into Europe by way of Arab traders coming to Venice. Venetian sailors then distributed the spice throughout the continent. Today, cloves are utilized in many dishes and in spicing drinks. Oil of cloves is commonly used as a breath freshener and to reduce gum pain, and has been used historically by herbalists to reduce nausea and stop vomiting.

Coriander (Coriandrum sativum): The seeds of coriander are used in curries and chili powder. The leaves of the plant are known as cilantro (see above).

Cumin Seed (Cuminum cyminum): This potent seed is an essential ingredient in curry powders as well as a basic seasoning in numerous Mexican, Indian, Spanish, and Middle Eastern recipes. It is a recognizable spice in humus, babaganoush, and other Middle Eastern dishes.

Curry Powder: Curry is not an individual spice but rather a blend of many different spices, often including cumin, cayenne, cloves, ginger, coriander, and turmeric. Generally in East Indian and Caribbean dishes, it brings a warm, spicy quality to any cuisine. Each culture has a different approach to creating curry mixtures. In India, curry is created with as many as ten herbs and spices. In Thailand, curry is used in conjunction with fresh herbs to give it a more delicate flavor.

Most serious cooks will mix their own curry combination, but you can purchase a mild curry blend for that delicious curry flavor without too much spiciness. If you are on a weight-management program and want to increase the thermogenic effect of curry, I recommend hot curry powder. It will make you sweat a little, but it will also increase your metabolism.

Masala is a curry-like powder that is commonly used in East Indian and Pakistani dishes. Unlike curry, Masala contains no turmeric and is sweeter than traditional curry powders.

Dandelion Root (Taraxacum officinale): A member of the daisy family native to Europe, dandelion is cultivated for both its leaves and roots. It is a perennial. The leaves can be included in a salad or cooked and served as a vegetable. The roots and rhizomes, when ground, can be used to flavor stimulant beverages such as coffee. Dandelion roots contain no caffeine. A mildly laxative and diuretic tea can be made from dandelion leaves. Dandelion promotes the formation of bile and, more generally, aids all secretion and excretion processes. Liver conditions such as gallstones and jaundice often respond to an infusion of dandelion root. Dandelions are a good source of calcium, iron, vitamin C, and beta-carotene.

Dill (Anethum graveolens): A member of the parsley family that is native to Europe, this annual plant is widely cultivated for its fruit, stems, leaves, and seeds. Dill is commonly used for its distinctive flavoring. Dill seed is a favorite herb, especially in traditional French and Middle Eastern cooking. French recipes for sauces, cakes, and pastries often contain dill seed.

Dill is also a popular spice in various pickled vegetables, especially cucumbers. Dill is derived from the old Norse word *dilla,* meaning "to lull." Many herbalists I know recommend dill seed tea to relieve colic in babies and for making a restful bedtime tea. I use dill seed most often in my cold salad dishes, especially coleslaw and potato and pasta salad.

Dill leaves and stems are a smoother, less pungent tasting version of dill seed. This culinary spice is used in various vegetable, dairy, tofu, and tempeh dishes.

Dill tea is a carminative (that is, it helps to break up intestinal gas) and has been used historically to treat upset stomachs.

Fennel Seeds (Foeniculum vulgare): These aromatic tasty seeds add a refreshing flavor to herbal and spice blends. In cookery, they can be substituted for dill and anise. I use fennel seeds in various sauces and Italian dishes. I often see fennel served in Indian restaurants at the end of the meal mixed with grated coconut. My friends tell me it helps reduce after dinner flatulence and also makes digestion easier after a heavy meal.

Fenugreek Seeds (Trigonella foenum-graecum): Whole fenugreek seeds are used in curries in India and as a condiment in Egypt. They also make a pleasing and tangy tea. Fenugreek seeds are one of the key ingredients in what many herbalists call the "liver flush." This formula is designed to support weight loss and general internal cleaning as the name implies by cleaning toxins out of the liver.

Garlic (Allium sativum): Garlic has been praised by many through the ages, including the Phoenicians and the Vikings, who carried large amounts of it on their sea voyages to strengthen and maintain their health. Traditionally known for the zest it adds to many cuisines, especially Italian, this favorite culinary spice is now available granulated, powdered, and minced. Garlic may be used in any dish. In weight reduction, garlic is valuable because it helps reduce undesirable types of cholesterol.

Ginger (Zingiber officinale): Along with garlic and peppermint, ginger is probably the most widely used herb in the world. It is frequently imported from China and West Africa. It adds a wonderfully robust flavor to all dishes and can be used as a food for hundreds of healing applications such as reducing fevers, digestive problems, and dizziness. It has thermogenic properties that make it a valuable herb for inclusion in weight-loss programs. In China, ginger and garlic are often added to a classic five-spice powder. This gives their food its distinctive quality. In the Caribbean, ginger is taken as a tea. Crystallized ginger is used in baking, Asian recipes, dips, and beverages including ginger tea, ginger ale, and non-alcoholic ginger beer. Ground ginger is often used in pickling blends and baked goods.

Jalapeno Peppers: These are green peppers used in Mexican cooking that are very hot. If I want real excitement, I'll add these to my tofu, seitan, and tempeh dishes.

Kelp (Fucus vesiculosis): This seaweed, or sea vegetable, provides a high source of minerals, including iodine, iron, and copper. It can be used as a tenderizer when cooking beans and as a salt substitute although it is not low in sodium. It can be used as an accent in soups, salads, and breads. In small quantities it may also be used as a salt substitute. It provides a high source of minerals, including iodine, iron, and copper. In small quantities, powdered kelp is often used as a salt substitute. The naturally occurring iodine found in kelp and other sea vegetables may slightly stimulate the thyroid gland, thus increasing metabolism and assisting in weight loss.

Lemongrass (Cymbopogon citratus): Frequently found in Thai, Vietnamese, and Chinese cooking, this tasty herb is also a key ingredient in Indonesian curries. In addition, lemongrass makes a relaxing tea.

In Asian cuisine, especially Indonesian cooking, flavor preferences tend to be sweet and sour. These flavors are achieved using lemongrass, tamarind, Kaffir lime, and various chilies.

Lemon Peel: A delightfully fresh-tasting herb for sauces, dessert frostings, and many entrees and baking, lemon peel also acts as a zesty ingredient in potpourris. Use only the peel from organically grown lemons.

Mace (Myristica fragans): Derived from the outside covering of nutmeg, mace is a favorite flavoring agent in eastern India in baking and cooking. Mace has a slightly stronger taste than nutmeg and is sometimes used as a substitute for it.

Marjoram (Majorana hortensis): The fragrance of this plant gives it its name, which means "joy of the mountain." Sweet marjoram, as it is also called, is an excellent seasoning to keep on hand for cooking a variety of vegetable dishes. I add it with garlic to flavor portobello mushrooms and tempeh dishes.

Mustard Seeds (Brassica nigra, Brassica juncea): Used since ancient times as a medicine and cooking spice, black mustard seeds are an essential ingredient in East Indian dishes. The more common yellow mustard seeds are used in pickling vegetables and making relishes, curries, and salads. The type of mustard that is spread on sandwiches comes from a combination of ground mustard seeds, vinegar, salt, and water.

Nutmeg (Myristica fragans): This widely used spice offers a warm and aromatic addition to your favorite hot or cold beverage. Nutmeg is especially popular in pumpkin pies and holiday dishes. The holiday-season smell that you may be familiar with is the smell of nutmeg.

Onion (Alluim cepa): A unique spice commonly used together with garlic, onion can be found in many cuisines. It is extremely versatile and takes on different tastes and textures depending on the type of onion used and whether it is cooked or used raw. Onion may be used fresh or granulated. It may be used on any dish especially salads, vegetables, soups, and sauces. Vidalia onions have a sweet taste, and are great on low-fat vegetable hero sandwiches. Onions thin the blood and lower cholesterol.

Orange Peel (Citrus aurantium): This culinary spice adds flavor to tofu, seitan and tempeh dishes, and baked goods. In addition, orange peel makes a delightful tea. But only use the peel of organically grown oranges.

Oregano (Origanum vulgare): An invaluable culinary spice, oregano is integral to many Italian and Mexican dishes especially those containing tomato sauce. It also makes a stimulating tea.

Parsley Leaves (Petroselinum crispum): The Greeks obviously held parsley in high esteem since they crowned their winning athletes with it. Though parsley has often been relegated to the side of the dish in burger restaurants, parsley leaves are often used by accomplished cooks to garnish and flavor a wide variety of foods including sauces, soups, salads, and tofu, tempeh, and seitan dishes. In Europe, the classic French herb combination includes parsley, chervil, and tarragon, among others.

Parsley and cracked wheat are the main ingredients in tabouleh, the popular Middle Eastern grain salad. Parsley is rich in vitamin C, vitamin A, calcium, magnesium, phosphorus, and potassium. Parsley tea is especially valued among herbalists for its diuretic properties and for the way it aids the adrenal and thyroid glands, which helps reduce water weight and increases metabolism.

Peppercorns: All peppers are not the same or even from the same botanical family. There are many types of pepper and they form one of the most popular and important groups of spices in cookery around the globe. Most peppers originate as peppercorns in India and are ground and packaged for commercial consumption. However, they can be purchased as whole peppercorns as well. The most popular peppercorns are white, black, and red. White peppercorns are fairly mild. I use them in light-colored sauces. Black peppercorns are generally hot to the taste. I use these in salads, soups, and dips. Red crushed peppercorns have a spicy taste. I like to add them to Italian dishes, especially my homemade low-fat pita pizza. Pepper is valuable for weight-loss programs due to its thermogenic properties.

Poppy Seed (Papaver somniferum): The delicate blue-black variety of this seed is a common cooking ingredient used to accent cakes, pastries, breads, and cakes.

Psyllium Seed (Plantago psyllium): These seeds are used to add bulk to the diet and as a stool-softener for those who suffer from constipation. They are often added to breakfast cereals and there are some brands of breakfast cereal that already contain psyllium.

Rosemary (Rosmarinus officinalis): The Latin name *rosmarinus* means "dew of the sea." This herb adds a light, pungent flavor to many cooked dishes. I use it in my herbed breads and in soups. It also adds a nice flavor to seitan, tofu, and tempeh dishes.

Saffron (Crocus sativus): Considered to be the gourmet cook's delight, saffron adds a delicate flavor and a rich golden hue to many dishes. It is commonly used in Indian cooking. This delicate spice is handpicked from the stigma of a unique type of crocus. Approximately forty-three hundred flowers are necessary for each ounce of saffron produced, so it can be quite costly. I use saffron in grain and pasta dishes as well as tofu, tempeh, seitan, meat, and vegetables dishes.

Sage (Salvia officinale): The name comes from a Latin word meaning "to be well." A member of the mint family, sage is also known as "red sage" or "garden sage." It has been used for centuries both in folk medicine and in the making of cosmetics. Today it is often added to stews, stuffing, sauces, and soups.

Savory (Satureja hortensis): The warm, peppery flavor of this herb is especially tasty when combined with marjoram and thyme. I know chefs and cooks who grow it fresh right in their little kitchen garden. It is my favorite herb for stuffing, and I use it in rice and millet dishes as well as in herb breads.

Shallots (Allium ascalonicum): Shallots are one of the milder members of the onion family. They add a subtle flavor to soups, sauces, and salads, and are a popular ingredient in many French recipes.

Spearmint (Mentha spicata): Alone or blended with other herbs, spearmint makes a highly refreshing drink. I like heating fresh spearmint in pineapple juice and then refrigerating it. Wow! Spearmint also adds a delectable freshness to vegetable dishes.

Sorrel (Rumex acetosa): Rich in iron, magnesium, phosphorus, sulfur, and silicon, sorrel is commonly used in Caribbean cooking and as a key ingredient in summer coolers.

Tamarind (Tamarindus indica): This sour fruit is commonly used instead of lemon juice in Middle Eastern, Indian, and Spanish cooking. It also makes a refreshing summer-winter drink called tamarindi. I boil the tamarind and add a little cinnamon, maple syrup, and ice cubes.

Tarragon (Artemisia dracunculus): Also called "little dragon," tarragon is a delicious culinary herb and an essential ingredient in the preparation of tarragon vinegar. I use it in salads, dressings, and breads.

Thyme (Thymus vulgaris): Thyme is considered a must in many stews, soups, salads, and stuffing. Thyme oil is used extensively in herbal medicine to reduce fevers and kill infections.

Turmeric (Curcuma longa): This spice gives many dishes a deep golden-yellow color and is an essential ingredient in curry powders and mustards. Indigenous to India, China, and the East Indies, turmeric is a member of the ginger family. I like to call turmeric the poor man's saffron. Because saffron is so costly, turmeric is often used as an inexpensive alternative for adding a mellow, yellow coloring to a dish. It is great for any dish where a yellow garnish is desired, including soups, stews, pickles, and relishes. I use turmeric in my tofu-based eggless egg salad.

Vanilla Bean (Vanilla planifolia, Vanilla tahitunsis): This fragrant bean is a popular addition to foods, desserts, and drinks. Brew a pot of coffee substitute with a small bit of vanilla bean. Sugar-free vanilla extract as well as fresh vanilla beans are available in natural food stores and spice shops. It is usually used in beverages, cakes, and other desserts.

Coffee, Tea, Cocoa

Most people don't realize that coffee, tea, and cocoa are actually herbal products. My suggestion is to avoid coffee and cocoa and use green tea instead. There are many reasons for this recommendation, but the main one is the caffeine and other naturally occurring chemicals found in coffee and cocoa products. These chemicals include theophyline, theobromine, and methylxanthine. Don't become disheartened. There are a number of safe and healthy alternatives to highly caffeinated beverages. Here are a few alternatives.

- *Coffee Substitutes*—There are many pleasant-tasting coffee substitutes available in supermarkets and health-food stores. If you have been a long-time coffee drinker you will find that these may take some getting used to, but there is a solution to this dilemma. Rather than eliminating coffee altogether you can start out with 50 percent of each and slowly decrease the coffee. In a few week's time you should be 100 percent coffee-free.

- *Tea*—In recent years the choices of caffeine-free teas has expanded to a point where you could probably drink a different flavor every day for a month. There are also some caffeine-free pekoe teas available and these are acceptable, though herbal tea such as chamomile, peppermint, or other choices are superior.

- *Cocoa*—It is unfortunate that cocoa contains caffeine and theobromine because chocolate treats like chocolate milk and hot chocolate are very popular with small children. Chocolate is also very high in fat, which is one of the reasons that it has such a smooth, rich texture. In recent years many people have begun to replace cocoa and chocolate with a wholesome and tasty powder made from the carob fruit. Carob has much less fat than sugar- and cocoa-derived products and is higher in fiber as well. Below is a recipe for a carob beverage that can be taken hot as a replacement for cocoa or cold as a shake:

Hot or Cold Carob
Ingredients:
>2 Tbsp. carob
>¼ cup sunflower oil (Olive oil would have too strong
>   a taste for this recipe)
>6 cups of rice or soy beverage
>4 tsp. of honey (or barley malt syrup)
>4 tsp. vanilla

Preparation Instructions:
Dissolve the carob powder in oil, add a rice or soy beverage, and heat the mixture for a few minutes to cook the carob. Place the mixture in a blender with the rest of the ingredients until it is smooth. Serve hot or refrigerate. This yields four to six servings.

Herbal Tea
>*Ingredients:*
>1 Tbsp. mullein leaves
>1 Tbsp. spearmint leaves
>¾ Tbsp. rose hips
>¾ Tbsp. orange peel
>A pinch of goldenseal

Preparation Instructions:
Boil water, pour over herb mixture, and steep for at least three minutes.

If you have an herb store or a well-stocked health-food store in your area, you can add other herbs with specific detoxification properties to your tea. Try buckthorn bark for constipation, fenugreek seeds for sore throats, coltsfoot for lung expectoration, papaya leaves for digestive upsets, blackberry root for diarrhea, or lemongrass for taste.

The above recipe is good for two to four cups of tea. The tea's effectiveness depends on its strength, and, of course, the greater the amount of water, the weaker the tea. Strong tea will be brown and weak tea will be yellow.

As you will note, the basic recipe calls for greater amounts of mullein and spearmint, and lesser amounts of orange and rose hips, which have strong flavors. Add only a small amount of goldenseal, as it is bitter and not very pleasing to the taste. But do not omit it as it is very important to the blend.

To make a large amount of the tea, you can add the rose hips to the water as it approaches boiling and the orange peel and leaves as the brew actually boils. Then turn the heat off, as you do not want the volatile elements of the leaves to evaporate. Let the mixture steep for two to three minutes, then strain. The leftover herbs can be used again for a weaker tea or a smaller pot.

You can prepare one cup of tea at a time by putting the appropriate herb amounts into a strainer and pouring boiling water over them directly into a cup. Let the strainer sit for a couple of minutes before removing it. You can make another cup or two of weaker tea from what's left in the strainer. The formula itself can be varied according to taste and availability of the herbs. Drink this tea consistently throughout the thirty-day program.

Chapter 9

The Thirty-Day Herbal

Weight-Loss Program

Introduction:

The introduction will tell you how to store spices and herbs and gives tips on herbal sprouting, steaming, broiling, baking, and frying.

Five Benefits from Using Herbs and Spices

1. They help reduce the salt and sugar content of your food.
2. They contain purifying properties.
3. They offer high flavor with little or no fat.
4. They are virtually calorie free.
5. They create greater variety in your purifying program.

Storing Herbs and Spices

I like to use fresh herbs and spices whenever it is possible, but sometimes I have to use the dried variety. Organically grown herbs and spices can sometimes be found in a supermarket, and are generally available in a wide variety in your local natural-food store.

When you store culinary herbs and spices, they should be kept in a dry, cool place with minimum exposure to sunlight and air. Bright light, heat, exposure to air, or the activity of fungi, plant enzymes, or bacteria may destroy herbal flavors and aromas.

I will sometimes buy fresh herbs and then store them by drying or freezing. If you are using fresh herbs and wish to store them, drying or freezing them are both effective approaches.

There are a number of ways to dry fresh herbs. My favorite is to lightly brush any dirt or other matter away using a pastry brush, but no water. Lay the herbs out in a dry, warm place on a screen or other airy surface. The herbs should dry in about a week and can then be stored in tinted, airtight glass jars. With some herbs, particularly bay leaves, the drying process actually improves the flavor of the herb.

With highly aromatic herbs, it is best to dry the fresh herbs in bundles. Gather a small bunch of herbs and brush any dirt or other matter away using a pastry brush, but no water. Tie them together with string or with a rubber band. Now hang the bunch upside down from a rack in a dry, cool area, with low humidity that does not exceed 86°F. This is important because a warmer environment will cause the essential oils of the herbs to evaporate. Because of all the cooking that goes on in a kitchen, this is not the best place to dry herbs.

If you wish, you can also dry fresh herbs by placing them in a brown paper bag. Label the bag so you will know what is in it, and place the bag in a cool, dry, dark place. Shake the bag every few days so the herbs dry evenly. Remove any stems, and crush the leaves or chop them into small pieces. Always store the dried herbs in tinted, airtight glass jars.

Note: when buying herbs and spices, seek out those that are organically grown and grown from non–genetically modified seeds.

Freezing Herbs
The herbs that store well with freezing are parsley, dill, fennel, and basil. Brush any dirt or other matter away using a pastry brush, but no water, then place about two or three tablespoons of each herb in separate freezer bags. Remember to label the bags.

Herb Sprouting
The best way to get fresh organically grown herbal greens is by growing your own sprouts. Sprouts are low in calories, rich in essential enzymes, nutrients, and chlorophyll, and easy to grow at

home. There are many types of sprouting seeds. The most popular are alfalfa, chickpea, lentil, mung bean, and sunflower.

1. Buy organically grown sprouting herb seeds at a health-food store. Place two tablespoons of sprouting seeds in a wide-mouthed quart container. Fill it with warm distilled water and cover the container with cheesecloth held by a rubber band. Soak overnight.

2. Every morning and evening for the next three to five days, drain the water from the jar using the cheesecloth as a strainer. Rinse with fresh distilled water, swirling sprouting material around. Drain again and place the jar in a warm place. Keep the sprouting material moist, but not wet, or it may rot. If your sprouts dry out between rinsing, top them with a moist white cotton towel or cheesecloth.

3. Harvest sprouts after three to five days or when they taste best to you.

Healthy Herbal Home Cooking

Adding herbs to broiled, baked, or steamed vegetables is an important part of the herbal weight-loss program. I recommend using commercial, non-fat, nonstick vegetable sprays. Many people like to lightly steam vegetables because steaming enables you to lightly cook vegetables without the use of butter or oil and, since most vegetables contain plenty of natural sodium, steamed vegetables require very little added salt. Once you add herbs to your vegetable dishes, you have great taste, herbal aromas, and great texture in your meals that keep them low in fat and interesting.

The most basic steamer to work with is the traditional bamboo steamer. This is a wonderful weight-management tool that can be found in many oriental supply stores. When using this multilevel-style steamer, remember that food cooks more rapidly in the bottom level. Remember to rotate the layers or put foods that take longer to cook in that bottom level.

If you are unable to find a bamboo steamer at your local store, you can use the common collapsible stainless steel steamer instead.

Caution: Remember that steam can burn, so tilt the lid away from you as you remove it. Don't allow the water level to drop too low or you may burn the pot and wind up with burnt-tasting vegetables.

Beans: Great Nutrition, Low in Fat and Calories

Beans (also called legumes) are a low-fat, fiber-rich food that are generally a good source of protein, and also contain minerals and B-vitamins. Most beans lack some of the key essential amino acids. For this reason, it is best to combine these foods with a grain whenever possible. The most popular and easily available beans are: adzuki beans, black beans, black-eyed peas, butter beans, chickpeas (garbanzo beans), green beans, kidney beans, lentils, lima beans, fava beans, navy/white beans, lima beans, pinto beans, soy beans, split peas, peanuts (yes, they really are legumes).

The Simple Way to Buy Beans

- Most dried legumes are available in see-through packages or in bulk. Whenever possible, buy them organically grown.
- Size—Look for a package with beans of uniform size. Small beans cook faster than large ones, and a variety of sizes will result in uneven cooking, causing large beans to be soft while the small ones will break up and become mushy.
- Color—Dried beans should have a bright, uniform color. Fading color is an indication that the bean has been in storage too long. Older beans take longer to cook and can be tasteless.
- Look for bags of beans that are free of any visible defects. These can include discoloration, cracked coating, foreign materials, perforations, and tears in the package itself.

Storing Beans: all dry, edible legumes are best stored in closed airtight containers in a cool, dry place or refrigerated. This will maintain the nutritional quality of the food and also reduce pest infestation.

How to Prepare Beans

A traditional way to use beans is to cook them for soup. They are great as refried beans and can be added to salads and casseroles. When mashed with spices and breadcrumbs, they make wonderful bean cakes. Most beans can be prepared by soaking them overnight in four times as much water as beans, and heating them for one and one half hours or until tender. In a pressure cooker, use water to cover the beans and cook for about twenty minutes at full pressure.

Seven Simple Steps for Cooking Beans

1. Always cook the beans in the water they were soaked in. If the beans begin to stick to the pot, add more water. Always keep the heat low. Beans that are cooked on a high flame will begin to break up, become mushy, and burn onto the pot.
2. Slightly undercook the beans if you are going to reheat them later. When you reheat them, they will be tender but still hold their shape. If you intend to puree or mash the beans, they should be cooked until they are very soft. Most beans require two to three hours of cooking. The exception is split peas and lentils. They will be tender in about forty-five minutes.
3. When preparing a recipe using beans, salt should be added last since salt hardens most beans and increases their cooking time. Add spices last as well, since the heat will dissipate the aroma and flavor of the oils.
4. Remember that beans expand when they cook. One cup of dry beans (approximately half a pound) will yield two to three cups after cooking. Be sure that you use a stainless steel pot large enough to accommodate this expansion.
5. Rinse the beans in filtered or distilled water.
6. Dried beans and whole peas should be soaked before cooking to replace water lost in drying and to reduce cooking time. Lentils and split peas are the exception to this rule. Most beans should be soaked in four times their

volume of water overnight. A quick-cook method is to bring the beans and water to a boil and then cook them for two minutes. Remove the beans from the heat, cover them, and let them soak for two hours. When you have finished soaking them, bring the beans and water to a boil, reduce to a very low heat, cover, and simmer gently until they are tender. This should take about two hours.

Soyfoods

In the last thirty years, the use of soybeans and soybean-based products (soyfoods) has exploded onto the American marketplace. This expanding popularity of soyfoods in the United States has come largely through the increase of interest in vegetarianism, macrobiotics, and Oriental cooking styles, as well as recent studies that show that soy products can reduce the risk of heart disease and cancer. Among the versatile, tasty, and low-fat soyfoods most commonly available are soy nuts, grits, flour, tempeh, tofu, lecithin, meat substitutes (tofu-based vegetarian hot dogs and luncheon meats like bologna, turkey etc.), TVP (textured vegetable protein), and dairy-free "soy" ice cream.

I recommend that individuals on a weight-management program seek out new protein substitutes, especially those that can mimic the texture and taste of animal foods such as eggs, chicken, beef, or meat. Beans fit the build in this department.

Tofu

Tofu, a bland, custard-like food made from soybeans, is the most popular and versatile of all of the soyfoods. A complete protein containing all eight essential amino acids, tofu is also rich in vitamins, minerals, fatty acids, and chemicals called phytoestrogens, which are believed to fight cancer as well as some of the difficult symptoms of menopause. Tofu is very low in saturated fat and has no cholesterol. It is attractive to cooks because it will take on the flavor of whatever food it's combined with.

More good news about tofu: it contains genistein, a compound some researchers think is a powerful cancer preventive. More women are now being urged to eat tofu as a replacement for hormone therapy for menopause. Tofu is valuable for men also. Research indicates that the same estrogen compounds that benefit women may help men stave off prostate cancer.

Because of its versatility, tofu is gaining increasing popularity as a high-quality vegetable protein source, especially for those looking to lose weight.

If you want to stay away from eggs, scramble up some tofu instead. If you want to be off meat for a while, or forever, add tofu to rice and vegetable. Make your chili with it. Put it in minestrone. I love to add it to my pasta dishes and pilafs. If we remain ignorant about this amazingly healthy food, it is our loss.

I often add dill, garlic, onion, and a little salt to create an herbed tofu spread. Mixed with other ingredients, tofu can be prepared to look like hot dogs, sausage, or cream cheese. In its basic form, tofu is generally sold either loose or in plastic, sealed, water-filled tubs and comes in three textures: soft, firm, and extra-firm. Each of these is used in different recipes.

Tempeh

Tempeh is a fermented soy product that is a staple food in Indonesia. It has become increasingly popular in the United States, and is sold as an eight-ounce, flat, rectangular patty. Tempeh is made through a multistep process that involves soaking, dehulling, and boiling. The beans are then mixed with a starter culture (a piece of tempeh from a previous batch) and a grain such as millet or brown rice. It is made much the way that a new batch of yogurt can be made by adding live yogurt culture to milk.

Tempeh can be used as a meat substitute and can be baked, steamed, boiled, or grilled. Tempeh is less versatile than tofu since tempeh has a strong distinctive taste and thus cannot be blended into other foods as easily. However, it is even more nutritionally balanced than tofu since it has live cultures and, unlike tofu, can be made from soybeans mixed with other cereal grains. You can find tempeh made from soy and millet, barley, or rice. This soy grain combination increases the protein value of tempeh without increasing the fat or calorie content. Fresh tempeh has the aroma of fresh-baked bread and a rich, earthy taste—sort of a cross between nuts and mushrooms. Tempeh is available at your local natural-food store.

Grains

Grains are intimately involved in the culture as well as the food and economy of many societies. Grains are an integral part of the creation myth of many cultures. For instance, according to Shinto belief, the Emperor of Japan is the living embodiment of *Ninigo-no-mikoto*, the god of the ripened rice plant.

The origin of grain has been debated for some time, but its uses are so ancient that the precise time and place of its first development will probably never be known. What is certain, however, is that the domestication of grain ranks as one of the most important developments in history. Grains have fed more people over a longer period of time than any other food.

Why are grains such nutritional powerhouses? Whole grains are rich in fiber, vitamins, minerals, and protein. Within each whole-grain berry or kernel, nature has packed all of the elements necessary to reproduce life. So long as it remains intact in this form, it will keep indefinitely. Among the most popular grains are amaranth, barley, corn, millet, wheat, oats, rice, quinoa, rye, buckwheat groats, and wild rice. Buckwheat is often incorrectly thought to be a member of the grass family, but it is actually a herbaceous plant from an entirely different botanical family. The fruits are commonly called buckwheat groats and may be ground into a flour or cooked and used as a cereal or a porridge, which is call kasha.

A whole grain contains the germ, endosperm, and bran, an incredible nutritional storehouse. Most grain-based foods that we are most familiar with are refined, that is to say that they have been stripped of the bran, and often of the germ as well. The germ is a rich source of vitamins E, B, and A, protein, and essential, unsaturated fatty acids. The endosperm is the part of the grain most familiar to Americans, because it is what remains after the bran and the germ have been processed out after the milling. It is a source of complex carbohydrates and virtually nothing else of importance to health. Most of us see the endosperm in the form of unbleached white flour.

In the last few years we have heard a lot about the value of bran, especially wheat and oat bran. Wheat bran was publicized as a source of fiber that could reduce colon cancer. Then the media publicized some studies that indicated that oat bran could reduce cholesterol levels. When taken as part of a whole grain, bran is a valuable source of nutrition. This outermost part of the grain is a source of fiber as well as B vitamins, proteins, fats, and minerals. Raw, unprocessed bran is recognized for its ability to promote the speedy movement of food wastes through the bowel, as well as help maintain stable blood sugar levels. Some bran is better than no bran, but a whole-grain cereal with the bran intact is the best choice.

Preparation: each grain will require a different approach to preparation. For instance, oats are often crushed to make oatmeal; wheat may be shredded in order to create the popular breakfast cereal or cracked in order to make the basis for tabouleh. Couscous is made from coarsely ground durham wheat (semolina) that has been precooked.

Generally grains appear as small hard "berries." Cook these berries using two parts water to one part grain, and cook for one to two hours. Most grains contain B vitamins, vitamin E, protein, iron, and several minerals.

When storing grains, keep them in a cool, dry place that is away from pests. Some grains will store up to three years; however, ground or processed flour, pancake mixes, etc., should be refrigerated and used frequently to maintain freshness.

The Basic Thirty-Day Program

Now I will show you day-by-day and step-by-step how to combine herbal strategies (Western herbs, Eastern herbs, Aromatherapy, Bach Remedies) as you plan your breakfasts, lunches, and dinners, starting with Day 1 of the Herbal Weight-Loss Program and ending with Day 30. All of these simple sample meal plans will affect the body's ability to shed weight in a progressive manner by balancing the essential nutrients while increasing metabolism with herbs. (An herbal/food grocery list for the week can be found at the end of the chapter.)

The Food Pyramid

Most nutritional consultants design food programs based on some form of the nutritional pyramid. In 1991-92 the USDA (United States Department of Agriculture) decided on a pyramid design that divided food groups into different levels telling us what we should eat the most of and what we should avoid. The placement of any one food in the pyramid was based on many factors, among them being their nutrient density and fat content.

The USDA pyramid, though an improvement over the four-food group structure that was used by mainstream nutritionists for many years, still has its problems. For instance, beans and meats are classified together, although they are very different in nutritional value and fat content. All dairy products are also classified together, although it's obvious that low-fat cottage cheese would be a more healthful choice than high-fat brie. Although grain products are the foundation of the pyramid, there is not a strong emphasis on whole grains as opposed to refined grain products.

To make my herbal weight-loss program more accessible, I have designed a nutritional pyramid structure specifically geared toward weight management. It uses the USDA pyramid as its basis, but a number of changes have been made to represent the specific focus of this book.

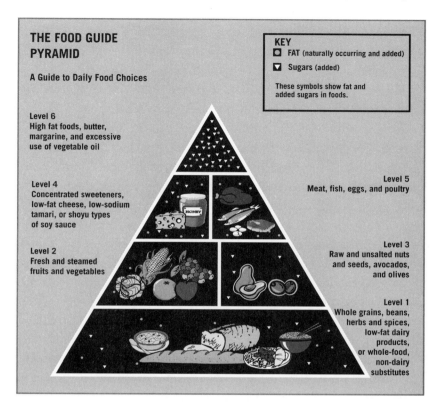

THE FOOD GUIDE PYRAMID

A Guide to Daily Food Choices

KEY
⬚ FAT (naturally occurring and added)
▽ Sugars (added)

These symbols show fat and added sugars in foods.

Level 6
High fat foods, butter, margarine, and excessive use of vegetable oil

Level 4
Concentrated sweeteners, low-fat cheese, low-sodium tamari, or shoyu types of soy sauce

Level 2
Fresh and steamed fruits and vegetables

Level 5
Meat, fish, eggs, and poultry

Level 3
Raw and unsalted nuts and seeds, avocados, and olives

Level 1
Whole grains, beans, herbs and spices, low-fat dairy products, or whole-food, non-dairy substitutes

Level 6:

High fat foods

Butter, margarine,

and excessive use of

vegetable oil

Level 5:

Meat, fish, eggs, and poultry

Level 4:

Concentrated sweeteners (honey,

maple syrup, molasses, brown sugar, dehydrated

cane and beet sugar), low-fat cheese,

low-sodium tamari, or shoyu types of soy sauce

Level 3:

Raw and unsalted nuts and seeds, nut and seed butters, avoca-

dos, and olives

219

Level 2:
Fresh and steamed fruits and vegetables
Level 1:
Whole grains, beans, herbs and spices, fermented, low-fat dairy products, or whole-food, non-dairy substitutes

Keys to the Herbal Weight-loss Pyramid

Level 6: High-fat foods. Avoid cream-based ice creams and sauces, butter, margarine, and large amounts of vegetable oil for cooking or in salad dressings. If you must use them, do so only occasionally. In spite of the recent popularity of high-fat, high-protein diets, most nutritional experts and researchers feel that a healthy diet based on complex carbohydrates and fruits and vegetables, with adequate protein and a balanced caloric intake, is the best dietary approach to weight loss.

Level 5: Meat, fish, eggs, and poultry. There are hundreds of diets that promote high-protein, high-fat, animal protein–based nutrition programs. Research indicates that, overall, a vegetarian-based program is the most nutritious and cost-effective approach to weight loss. If you feel that you require flesh foods as part of your dietary program, use egg whites or some fish as part of your transition from a diet high in meat or poultry.

Level 4: Concentrated sweeteners (honey, maple syrup, molasses, brown sugar, dehydrated cane and beet sugar), low-fat cheese, low-sodium tamari, or shoyu types of soy sauce. Sweeteners are a good source of flavoring for fruit desserts and smoothies, but should be used in moderation. Barley malt syrup is the most desirable. It is available in most health-food stores. Low-fat cheeses are a high source of calcium and protein, but also tend to be high in salt and may contain artificial colors or ingredients to mimic the texture and taste of regular whole-milk cheese products. When buying soy sauce, read the label in order to avoid benzoate preservatives that are used in lower quality products.

Level 3: Raw and unsalted nuts and seeds, nut and seed butters, avocados, and olives. These are high-value, healthy foods, but are of a higher fat content and higher caloric value than Level 1. They should be used regularly but in moderate amounts. These foods are as essential as those in Level 1, but also contain certain foods that supplement the foods in Level 1. Flaxseed oil, evening primrose oil, and olive oil are examples.

Level 2: Fruits and vegetables. These are rich in vitamins, minerals, fiber enzymes, and other key factors, especially antioxidants.

Level 1: This level consists of whole grains, beans, herbs, and foods made from them. Included are: whole-grain breads, grain- and soy-based milk substitutes, soy- and rice-based cheese substitutes, tofu- and grain-based deli meat substitutes (low in fat, free of nitrates and other artificial ingredients), low-fat, non-fat, and fermented milk products such as yogurt, kefir, cottage cheese, and buttermilk, and spices for flavoring foods. This is the largest and the primary structure of the program. Most of the essential nutrients—proteins, essential fatty acids, carbohydrates, vitamins, minerals, and fiber—are found on this level. The herbs can increase metabolism and cleanse the system.

Starting the Program

You are about to begin a journey of discovery. After you have launched yourself on this program, you will begin to realize that the improvements in your strength, vitality, endurance, moods, and general well-being are a reward that you could not have imagined.

Include lots of high-fiber foods and complex carbohydrates in your diet, such as fresh fruits, vegetables, whole grains, and beans. You may be pleased to learn that as much as 30 percent of the calories found in complex carbohydrates are not absorbed and will pass through your body without adding to your caloric intake.

Remember: avoid high-calorie foods, alcohol, foods with refined white sugar or brown sugar, too much sodium, foods with too much saturated fat, gravies, heavy sauces, and foods that are too hot or too cold. Also avoid drinking fluids excessively with your meals and eating when you are under great stress.

It Is Best To

- Broil, steam, or bake all foods that you do not eat raw. Do not add oil or butter. Use nonstick vegetable spray when necessary.
- Prepare small portions.
- Use only honey and maple syrup, in moderation, if you must use sweeteners at all.
- Use soy or rice milk instead of cow's milk if you must use milk.
- The best snacks are herbal teas or tofu cubes, celery sticks or fruit slices (apples, pears, etc.), and cottage cheese. As you become more successful, you can add peaches, plums, and mangos. Eat one or two snacks in the afternoon, and space them no farther than three hours apart. Spacing your snacks will balance your blood sugar and increase thermogenesis.
- Add thermogenic spices such as cayenne, mustard, and pepper to your foods. Also add lemon, cider vinegar, natural tamari soy sauce, and ketchup (homemade or from a natural-food store) to your foods if you like.

Motivate Yourself!

Let's face it, the truth is that if you are not sufficiently motivated, you will not lose weight. You must motivate yourself to a great degree, but you can also rely on others for added support. Learn to rely on your family, friends, and coworkers for help in keeping to your weight-loss program. Better yet, consider joining a weight-loss support group.

You must actively work to keep your motivation high. Here are a number of do's and don'ts to keep your motivation level at its peak:

1. Ask your family and friends not to entice you with food, snacks, treats, or anything else that can undermine your program. Control your home environment so you will be able to avoid factors that foster overeating, such as easy access to food and having food in full view.

2. Learn to choose the proper foods in restaurants, even though friends and associates may be eating foods that are not on your diet.

3. Don't accept food that has not been prepared as you requested in restaurants. Don't be shy; talk to the waiter or waitress, or, if necessary, the maitre d'.

4. Don't allow friends or acquaintances to sabotage your efforts (innocently or otherwise) by saying things such as, "You look fine—you don't really need to lose weight." You will want to agree, of course, but you must stand firm. Do not give in to such temptation.

5. Don't be embarrassed at parties or other social functions when you are asked why you are not eating certain foods. Answer truthfully. There is no shame in dieting.

6. Don't be "forced" into eating something by comments such as, "Try this—I just cooked it." Or "It's only a little piece—it won't hurt you." Politely decline.

7. Avoid watching tempting food commercials. Change the channel.

8. Learn to make eating a wonderful experience. After all, it is.

Putting It into Practice

As you put the daily meal plans into practice, notice that in the morning you can review how you feel emotionally and reduce the influence of emotional factors on overeating homeopathically with herbal flower remedies. Review your emotional state and use the appropriate herbal Bach Remedy twenty minutes after breakfast.

When your diet starts to change in following these rules, your intake of animal protein (meat, chicken, eggs, and milk products) will decrease. It will be replaced by many foods of vegetable origin that are not only rich in complex carbohydrates that will provide you with energy, but are also rich in protein.

We now know that even though many vegetable foods on their own do not contain all of the essential amino acids necessary to provide "complete protein," a combination of vegetable foods eaten together can. There are innumerable delicious combinations of vegetable foods that deliver perfect protein, minus the pesticides, antibiotics, hormones, and various other residues that all non-organically raised animal products carry with them, and little, if any, of the saturated fat in much animal food, organically raised or not.

This new diet will feed you well. It will be rich in vitamins, minerals, trace elements, enzymes, essential fatty acids, and essential amino acids. It will create greater well-being and health for you, and it will cost you less than what you're eating now.

I have spoken about protein and good, low-calorie protein sources throughout the book. The following foods are a reminder that there are many low-fat, good sources of complete protein. Some of them are animal and some are vegetable. I list them here to give you the assurance that it is relatively easy to find something to eat that will provide you with at least as much protein as a hamburger or a couple of eggs or pieces of chicken.

1. Yogurt, buttermilk, soy cheeses, and low-fat milk products
2. Tofu
3. Tempeh
4. Yeast—brewer's or nutritional
5. Micro algae

As much as possible, prepare your own meals. Many low-calorie foods contain synthetic flavorings and flavor enhancers (such as MSG). These chemicals have no nutritional value and serve only to mask the poor flavor quality of an overprocessed food. Many people have strong allergic reactions to MSG, giving all of us an additional reason to avoid this unnecessary additive.

Remember that our forebearers found that flavorings and spices made their foods more palatable, added variety to routine foods, and made mealtime a pleasure rather than a necessity. As you become familiar with our herbal recipes, you will discover how herbs and spices such as cinnamon, chili, and vanilla can make your healthy food a joy to prepare and serve.

For appetite appeal, it is important that foods have character-istic and attractive colors. In processing or cooking foods, changes occur that require the addition of a coloring agent to recapture the characteristic color.

People lose weight at different rates. Individual characteristics such as sex, age, activity level, and metabolic condition determine the rate at which fat is burned. For this reason the thirty-day menu can be adjusted to those with fast or slow metabolisms in order to jump-start the fat-eliminating process. There are three basic programs you can apply to the menu structure to maximize your fat burning potential.

Program 1: The Basic Meal Plan

The thirty-day menu structure is designed as a good starting point for beginners. This basic plan is based on main dishes consisting of various combinations of grains and beans. If this becomes bor-ing you can replace the grain/bean choices with entree recipes listed in the back of the book. These various recipes are built around combinations of proteins, carbohydrates, and vegetables. Start with the basic plan. These meals, combined with the herbal supplements and teas, will burn more calories each week. You should stay on Program 1 as you continue to lose body fat at a steady rate.

This is not designed to be a rigid program. The herbal sup-plements, teas, and extracts will increase your metabolism and fat-burning processes, while controlling your appetite and enhancing your energy. Many of these herbs help increase body metabolism (thermogenesis) so they will help your body convert ingested calories and stored fat into heat instead of fat. The food plans are arranged to balance blood-sugar levels, decrease appetite, lower cholesterol and triglycerides, inhibit fat synthesis, and diminish cravings.

As for the menus, any breakfast can be replaced by any other breakfast as long as the portions are the same. This also applies to the lunch and dinner menus.

If you do not want to use the main dish recipe choices I have included in the thirty-day program, then consider the basic low-fat, high-protein combinations and the herbed protein combos mentioned below instead.

1. Bean soup (lentil, lima, or pea, etc.), with nuts or seeds or rice or pasta added
2. Chili beans with corn tortillas
3. Whole-wheat bread with natural (100 percent peanut) peanut butter
4. Black-eyed peas and cornbread made with whole-wheat flour
5. Brown rice and beans

Herbed Protein Combos

1. Split pea soup with garlic and onions and whole-grain bread sticks
2. Tarragon-flavored black-eyed peas with corn bread
3. Whole-wheat bread and unsweetened natural peanut butter
4. Whole corn tortillas and low-fat refried beans and chili powder
5. Any bean soup (pea, lentil, lima bean, etc.) with sesame seeds or sunflower seeds added
6. Corn and bean salad with sage and tarragon
7. Red or black beans with sage and thyme and brown rice with powdered kelp

While on the thirty-day program, do not change or alter the herbal recommendations. Until you hit a plateau in your fat loss, you do not need to change the way that you are eating.

Snacks

A key factor in achieving success with Program 1 is to plan snacks that have healthy mini-meals of weight-loss promoting herb teas, and filling, low-fat foods. Try whole-grain cold cereal with a rice beverage, pretzels and low-fat yogurt, baked corn chips, low-fat granola, whole-grain pita pockets stuffed with vegetables and low-fat, natural salad dressing, fresh fruit and fresh vegetables dipped in low-fat herb dip, and best of all, water with lemon or soup with cayenne or other thermogenic spices added.

Program 2: For Those with 30 Percent Body Fat or More

You can measure your body fat level through a physician or from a trainer at a health club. If you have 30 percent body fat or more, you should be ready to move on to Program 2 after two weeks. This food plan differs from Program 1 in that here you are limiting your food intake to a bowl of broth and a large salad and eliminating carbohydrates from the evening meal. By reducing your carbohydrate consumption, you inhibit the release of insulin, which then stimulates glucagon, a hormone that helps to unlock fat.

Also, when carbohydrates are eliminated at night, fewer stored carbohydrates (glycogen) are available for energy the following morning. Without glycogen, your body burns fatty acids (stored body fat) for energy, thus accelerating fat loss. Doing aerobic exercise prior to breakfast can accelerate it even further. Then, when you consume carbohydrates at breakfast and lunch, they are efficiently synthesized into glycogen, are stored in the muscles, and are much less likely to turn into body fat.

When you eat in the evening try not to eat after 8 P.M. You may also use a thermogenic herbal formula oil to help burn fat and boost your metabolism.

After about three weeks, you may want to start adding starchy carbohydrates back into your evening meal. Try adding beans and legumes, which are high in protein and have a high metabolic effect.

Program 3: If You've Been Struggling With Dieting for Years

This program is designed for those whose metabolisms are truly slow and should only be followed for two or three days of the week. Only try this program if you've been a chronic dieter and have not lost a reasonable amount of body fat on Program 2. It is well-balanced nutritionally, but is restrictive and can get boring. Definitely stick to Program 1 if you have a history of yo-yo dieting or eating disorders.

While on Program 3, eliminate most carbohydrates after 3 P.M. Add a regular aerobic workout to your schedule, either in the morning, in the evening, or both. By doing this, you force your body to draw on its own stored fat for energy. You can still get the nutrition you need from lean proteins such as non-fat yogurt, low-fat cottage cheese, and firm tofu served in vegetable soup.

Also restrict food high on the glycemic index including potatoes, bread, raisins, carrots, and watermelon, and foods that rank as moderate on the glycemic index including most types of pasta, bulgur, baked beans, yams, green peas, sweet potatoes, orange juice, blueberries, and rice. Instead, eat plenty of soup, large salads, and plenty of steamed vegetables low on the glycemic index. (See glycemic index, pg. 106.)

As with Program 2, stick with high-protein beans and legumes as you add carbohydrates back into your diet or if you are hungry in the evening.

Use a thermogenic herbal formula with your meals. Thermogenic herbal formulas act as energy in your body, bringing it into fat-burning mode and increasing your metabolism.

Program 1: The Basic Meal Plan
Week One—Internal Cleaning

The basic goal of internal cleaning is to purify the body's internal ecosystem with herbs and remove toxic metabolic wastes and other clogging substances that have resulted from eating highly processed, denatured food, breathing poor air, drinking tainted water, and living under artificial light and emotional stress. The herbs used are the keys to restoring a nourishing environment in and around the body so that natural weight loss can begin. Here I have outlined a breakfast, lunch, and dinner menu for each of the thirty days. I have also included snacks and Bach Remedies, aromatherapy, and herbal supplement recommendations.

Note: be consistent with the herbal aspects of the program as well as with the dietary suggestions. Apply the herbal suggestions throughout the day. With twenty minutes of aerobic exercise daily, you may expect to lose from three to five pounds during week one.

(Warning: if you take our recommended herbal supplements *do not* drink coffee. You can overstimulate yourself.)

Week One Day 1

1. Do the ten-minute aromatherapy program upon awakening.
2. About ten minutes before breakfast and fifteen minutes after the completion of the aromatherapy program, have a six-ounce cup of licorice tea and four capsules of fiber-rich herbs.
3. Suggested breakfast: one cup of fresh fruit salad (include apples, pears, melon, and half a banana or cantaloupe). You may use a coffee substitute. A few available brand names include Roastarama, Pero, and Cafix.
4. Reduce the influence of emotional factors on overeating with Bach Remedies: ten minutes after breakfast, review your emotional state and use the appropriate herbal flower remedy.
5. Take Cleansing Tea ten minutes before lunch, either in capsule form or as a liquid extract. Place twenty drops of extract Buchu (Agathosma betulina) in a glass of warm water. This herb is a cleanser for the genito-urinary system.
6. Suggested lunch: a cup of lentil soup or clear vegetable broth, a small mixed green salad, and a cup of tofu, eggless egg salad.
7. Ten minutes before dinner have a six-ounce cup of parsley tea for kidney cleansing.
8. Remember: eat dinner by no later than 8 P.M., if possible. Try a cup of soup and my Tempeh Salad (see recipe) with thermogenic dressing.
9. Take two burdock capsules for liver cleansing ten minutes after dinner.

Week One Day 2

1. Do the ten-minute aromatherapy program upon awakening.
2. About ten minutes before breakfast and fifteen minutes after the completion of the aromatherapy program, have a six-ounce cup of licorice tea and four capsules of fiber-rich herbs.
3. Suggested breakfast: one cup oat bran with half a banana. You may use a coffee substitute. A few available brand names include Roastarama, Pero, and Cafix.
4. Reduce the influence of emotional factors on overeating with Bach Remedies: ten minutes after breakfast review your emotional state and use the appropriate herbal flower remedy.
5. Take Cleansing Tea ten minutes before lunch, either in capsule form or as a liquid extract. Place twenty drops of extract Buchu (Agathosma betulina) in a glass of warm water. This herb is a cleanser for the genito-urinary system.
6. Suggested lunch: a cup of split pea soup or clear vegetable broth, a small mixed green salad, and steamed spinach, broccoli, or cauliflower.
7. Ten minutes before dinner have a six-ounce cup of parsley tea for kidney cleansing.
8. Suggested dinner: buckwheat (soba) noodles with soft tofu, garlic, and herbs, and a small green salad.
9. Take two burdock capsules for liver cleansing ten minutes after dinner.

Week One Day 3

1. Do the ten-minute aromatherapy program upon awakening.
2. About ten minutes before breakfast and fifteen minutes after the completion of the aromatherapy program, have a six-ounce cup of licorice tea and four capsules of fiber-rich herbs.
3. Suggested breakfast: Spanish-style half tofu scramble with sautéed peppers, onions, and tomatoes (sautéed in non-fat spray). You may use a coffee substitute. A few available brand names include Roastarama, Pero, and Cafix.

4. Reduce compulsive eating with Bach Remedies: ten minutes after breakfast review your emotional state and use the appropriate herbal flower remedy.
5. Take Cleansing Tea ten minutes before lunch, either in capsule form or as a liquid extract. Place twenty drops of extract Buchu (Agathosma betulina) in a glass of warm water. This herb is a cleanser for the genito-urinary system.
6. Suggested lunch: a cup of onion soup (onions sautéed in 1 tsp. of olive oil and cooked with vegetable soup powder) or clear vegetable broth, a small mixed green salad, and half a cup of steamed or baked yams.
7. Ten minutes before dinner have a six-ounce cup of parsley tea for kidney cleansing.
8. Suggested dinner: one broccoli and garlic-stuffed baked potato (or half a cup of mashed, steamed Jerusalem Artichoke with 1 tsp. of olive oil and fresh chopped garlic), and a small green salad. One half whole-grain pita bread.
9. Take two burdock capsules for liver cleansing ten minutes after dinner.

Week One Day 4

1. Do the ten-minute aromatherapy program upon awakening.
2. About ten minutes before breakfast and fifteen minutes after the completion of the aromatherapy program, have a six-ounce cup of licorice tea and four capsules of fiber-rich herbs.
3. Suggested breakfast: one cup puffed, whole-grain cereal (wheat, corn, rice, or millet) with six ounces non-dairy soy or rice beverage. Or, have half a cantaloupe. You may use a coffee substitute. A few available brand names include Roastarama, Pero, and Cafix.
4. Reduce compulsive eating with Bach Remedies: ten minutes after breakfast review your emotional state and use the appropriate herbal flower remedy.
5. Take Cleansing Tea ten minutes before lunch, either in

capsule form or as a liquid extract. Place twenty drops of extract Buchu (Agathosma betulina) in a glass of warm water. This herb is a cleanser for the genito-urinary system.

6. Suggested lunch: a cup of mushroom and barley soup or clear vegetable broth, a small mixed green salad and steamed spinach, broccoli, or cauliflower.

7. Ten minutes before dinner have a six-ounce cup of parsley tea for kidney cleansing.

8. Suggested dinner: Italian Sloppy Joes (see recipe at back of book) on a whole-grain hamburger bun and a small mixed green salad.

9. Take two burdock capsules for liver cleansing ten minutes after dinner.

Week One Day 5

1. Do the ten-minute aromatherapy program upon awakening.

2. About ten minutes before breakfast and fifteen minutes after the completion of the aromatherapy program, have a six-ounce cup of licorice tea and four capsules of fiber-rich herbs.

3. Suggested breakfast: one slice of 100 percent whole-grain toast with unsweetened fruit spread, low-fat cottage cheese, or low-fat soy cream cheese. Or, have a cup of fresh fruit salad (include apples, pears, melon, and half a banana). You may use a coffee substitute. A few available brand names include Roastarama, Pero, and Cafix.

4. Reduce compulsive eating with Bach Remedies: ten minutes after breakfast review your emotional state and use the appropriate herbal flower remedy.

5. Take Cleansing Tea ten minutes before lunch, either in capsule form or as a liquid extract. Place twenty drops of extract Buchu (Agathosma betulina) in a glass of warm water. This herb is a cleanser for the genito-urinary system.

6. Suggested lunch: ten ounce Balanced Carbo-Protein Herbal Smoothie.

7. Ten minutes before dinner have a six-ounce cup of parsley

tea for kidney cleansing.

8. Suggested dinner: Mock Lasagna (see recipe at back of book) and a small green salad.

9. Take two burdock capsules for liver cleansing ten minutes after dinner.

Week One Day 6

1. Do the ten-minute aromatherapy program upon awakening.

2. About ten minutes before breakfast and fifteen minutes after the completion of the aromatherapy program, have a six-ounce cup of licorice tea and four capsules of fiber-rich herbs.

3. Suggested breakfast: twelve ounces of one of the Blended Drink Recipes.

4. Reduce compulsive eating with Bach Remedies: ten minutes after breakfast review your emotional state and use the appropriate herbal flower remedy.

5. Take Cleansing Tea ten minutes before lunch, either in capsule form or as a liquid extract. Place twenty drops of extract Buchu (Agathosma betulina) in a glass of warm water. This herb is a cleanser for the genito-urinary system.

6. Suggested lunch: a cup of mixed vegetable soup or clear vegetable broth, a small mixed green salad, and steamed broccoli.

7. Ten minutes before dinner have a six-ounce cup of parsley tea for kidney cleansing.

8. Suggested dinner: one cup of any steamed vegetable or combination of vegetables (broccoli, zucchini, kale, carrots, and yellow squash are good choices) and a cup of brown rice.

9. Take two burdock capsules for liver cleansing ten minutes after dinner.

Week One Day 7

1. Do the ten-minute aromatherapy program upon awakening.

2. About ten minutes before breakfast and fifteen minutes after the completion of the aromatherapy program,

have a six-ounce cup of licorice tea and four capsules of fiber-rich herbs.

3. Suggested breakfast: one cup of fresh fruit salad (include apples, pears, melon, and half a banana). Or, have half a cantaloupe. You may use a coffee substitute. A few available brand names include Roastarama, Pero, and Cafix.

4. Reduce compulsive eating with Bach Remedies: ten minutes after breakfast review your emotional state and use the appropriate herbal flower remedy.

5. Take Cleansing Tea ten minutes before lunch, either in capsule form or as a liquid extract. Place twenty drops of extract Buchu (Agathosma betulina) in a glass of warm water. This herb is a cleanser for the genito-urinary system.

6. Suggested lunch: a cup of chunky vegetable soup (broccoli, zucchini, mushrooms, potatoes, water, and powdered soup mix) or clear vegetable broth, a small mixed green salad, and brown rice.

7. Ten minutes before dinner have a six-ounce cup of parsley tea for kidney cleansing.

8. Suggested dinner: Scalloped Potatoes with Low-Fat Cottage Cheese and Herbs de Provence (see recipes in back of book), and a small green salad.

9. Take two burdock capsules for liver cleansing ten minutes after dinner.

Tips for Week One

- Read package labels or consult basic food-nutrient tables for fat content; keep track of grams of fat in your diet, and target areas that need work. Note: goals for fat intake apply to the diet over several days, not to a single meal or food. Balance is the overall key.

- One good way to lower the fat content of your diet is to modify the recipes you follow. Ask yourself these questions: can the fat be reduced? In baked goods, such as cookies, quick breads, and some cakes, substitute three-fourths of the fat called for with an equal amount of low-fat yogurt, applesauce, or prune puree. Make one cup of puree by blending eight ounces of dried prunes and six tablespoons of water in a food processor or blender. Rather than add additional oil to prepackaged cake and brownie mixes, substitute completely with applesauce or yogurt. Can you steam, boil, broil, or sauté with nonstick spray rather than fry?

- Internal cleansing as an approach to weight management is based on the idea that herbal body purification can assist in removing the metabolic causes of obesity. Under normal conditions your immune system, utilizing each organ of elimination, will maintain a healthy and balanced internal environment. Under the abnormal conditions of stress created by an unhealthy lifestyle and the intake of toxic substances, these organs become loaded with systemic poisons. This toxic overloading radically alters the internal ecosystem of your body, reducing the intake of essential nutrients and causing you to feel hungry and eat more, even though your daily caloric intake may already be high.

Week Two—An Asian Approach

The second week of the herbal program is based on a dietary and herbal program that synthesizes a multifaceted Asian approach to herbal weight loss. Combining Indian and Chinese herbs with a diet of grains, beans, salads, and special Asian herbal teas will help burn away fat and increase your metabolism.

Week Two Day 8

1. Do the ten-minute aromatherapy program upon awakening.
2. Take one cup of green tea five minutes before breakfast.
3. Suggested breakfast should consist of oatmeal, hot brown-rice cereal, or another whole-grain complex carbohydrate. Whole-grain cereals are great for quick energy. Add a protein, such as a soy shake, for a more lasting boost.

4. Reduce compulsive eating with Bach Remedies: ten minutes after breakfast review your emotional state and use the appropriate herbal flower remedy.
5. Take the Indian herb Garcinia cambogia in capsule form. This will reduce your appetite and help burn fat.
6. Suggested lunch: one cup of sautéed (use nonstick spray instead of oil) carrots, cabbage, peas, and corn. Serve with clear vegetable broth with scallions and four ounces of sliced tofu.
7. Ten minutes before dinner, take capsules of Siberian Ginseng.
8. Suggested dinner: Broiled Leeks with Herbed Vinaigrette and a cup of curried brown rice.
9. Have one cup of Gotu Kola Tea or green tea—to balance the nervous system before sleeping.

Week Two Day 9

1. Do the ten-minute aromatherapy program upon awakening.
2. Take one cup of green tea five minutes before breakfast.
3. Suggested breakfast: one cup of fresh fruit salad (include apples, pears, melon, and half a banana). Or, have half a cantaloupe. You may use a coffee substitute. A few available brand names include Roastarama, Pero, and Cafix.
4. Reduce compulsive eating with Bach Remedies: ten minutes after breakfast review your emotional state and use the appropriate herbal flower remedy.
5. Take the Indian herb Garcinia cambogia in capsule form. This will reduce your appetite and help burn fat.
6. Suggested lunch: one cup of carrot-yam soup, half of a whole-wheat pita, and one cup of a steamed, pleasant-tasting sea vegetable (arame, wakamae, kombu, hijiki, or nori).
7. Ten minutes before dinner, take capsules of Siberian Ginseng.
8. Suggested dinner: Herbed Chinese Seitan Nuggets and a small green salad.

9. Have one cup of Gotu Kola Tea or green tea—to balance the nervous system before sleeping.

Week Two Day 10
1. Do the ten-minute aromatherapy program upon awakening.
2. Take one cup of green tea five minutes before breakfast.
3. Suggested breakfast: half a cup whole-grain cereal with six ounces of soy milk or rice beverage.
4. Reduce compulsive eating with Bach Remedies: ten minutes after breakfast review your emotional state and use the appropriate herbal flower remedy.
5. Take the Indian herb Garcinia cambogia in capsule form. This will reduce your appetite and help burn fat.
6. Suggested lunch: one cup of sautéed (use nonstick spray instead of oil) carrots, cabbage, peas and corn. Serve with clear vegetable broth with scallions and four ounces sliced tofu.
7. Ten minutes before dinner, take capsules of Siberian Ginseng.
8. Suggested dinner: Scalloped Potatoes with Low-Fat Cottage Cheese and Herbs de Provence (see recipes in back of book), and a small green salad.
9. Have one cup of Gotu Kola Tea or green tea— to balance the nervous system before sleeping.

Week Two Day 11
1. Do the ten-minute aromatherapy program upon awakening.
2. Take one cup of green tea five minutes before breakfast.
3. Suggested breakfast: twelve ounces of one of the Blended Drink Recipes.
4. Reduce compulsive eating with Bach Remedies: ten minutes after breakfast review your emotional state and use the appropriate herbal flower remedy.
5. Take the Indian herb Garcinia cambogia in capsule form. This will reduce your appetite and help burn fat.

6. Suggested lunch: a cup of mixed vegetable soup or clear miso soup with three dim sum (vegetable dumplings from a health-food store), one cup of a steamed, pleasant-tasting sea vegetable (arame, wakamae, kombu, hijiki, or nori).
7. Ten minutes before dinner, take capsules of Siberian Ginseng.
8. Suggested dinner: Herbed Chinese Seitan Nuggets and a small green salad.
9. Have one cup of Gotu Kola Tea or green tea—to balance the nervous system before sleeping.

Week Two Day 12

1. Do the ten-minute aromatherapy program upon awakening.
2. Take one cup of green tea five minutes before breakfast.
3. Suggested breakfast: half a cup whole-grain cereal with six ounces of soy milk or rice beverage.
4. Reduce compulsive eating with Bach Remedies: ten minutes after breakfast review your emotional state and use the appropriate herbal flower remedy.
5. Take the Indian herb Garcinia cambogia in capsule form. This will reduce your appetite and help burn fat.
6. Suggested lunch: ten ounces of Balanced Carbo-Protein Herbal Smoothie.
7. Ten minutes before dinner, take capsules of Siberian Ginseng.
8. Suggested dinner: a grilled tofu sandwich. Grill or roast tofu, onions, and peppers, and serve them on whole-grain pita with mustard or low-fat salad dressing. Add lettuce, tomato, and pickles.
9. Have one cup of Gotu Kola Tea or green tea—to balance the nervous system before sleeping.

Week Two Day 13

1. Do the ten-minute aromatherapy program upon awakening.
2. Take one cup of green tea five minutes before breakfast.

3. Suggested breakfast: half a cup whole-grain cereal with six ounces of soy milk or rice beverage.
4. Reduce compulsive eating with Bach Remedies: ten minutes after breakfast review your emotional state and use the appropriate herbal flower remedy.
5. Take the Indian herb Garcinia cambogia in capsule form. This will reduce your appetite and help burn fat.
6. Suggested lunch: a cup of split pea soup or clear miso soup, a small mixed cabbage salad with rice vinegar, soy sauce, and a teaspoon of sesame oil mixed as a dressing, and half a cup grilled mushrooms with onions.
7. Ten minutes before dinner, take capsules of Siberian Ginseng.
8. Suggested dinner: a grilled tempeh and mushroom sandwich. Serve on a whole-grain pita with mustard or low-fat salad dressing. Add lettuce, tomato, and pickles and one cup of a steamed, pleasant-tasting sea vegetable (arame, wakamae, kombu, hijiki, or nori).
9. Have one cup of Gotu Kola Tea or green tea—to balance the nervous system before sleeping.

Week Two Day 14

1. Do the ten-minute aromatherapy program upon awakening.
2. Take one cup of green tea five minutes before breakfast.
3. Suggested breakfast: half a cup whole-grain cereal with six ounces of soy milk or rice beverage.
4. Reduce compulsive eating with Bach Remedies: ten minutes after breakfast review your emotional state and use the appropriate herbal flower remedy.
5. Take the Indian herb Garcinia cambogia in capsule form. This will reduce your appetite and help burn fat.
6. Suggested lunch: try a cup of soup and Curry Baked Tofu.
7. Ten minutes before dinner, take capsules of Siberian Ginseng.
8. Suggested dinner: a cup of mushroom and barley soup or

clear vegetable broth, a small mixed green salad and one cup of a steamed, pleasant-tasting sea vegetable (arame, wakamae, kombu, hijiki, or nori).

9. Have one cup of Gotu Kola Tea or green tea—to balance the nervous system before sleeping.

Tips for Week Two

- Beverages can include any variety of teas or grain drinks, including grain tea. Special macrobiotic teas, such as Mu tea or Bancha tea are available at your local health-food store.

- Use whole grains (brown rice, whole barley, millet, kasha). These are all available at your local market.

- Experiment with different types of beans. Try chickpeas, lentils, green peas, lima beans, or navy beans. They are inexpensive and when eaten with grains are a great source of complete protein.

- Each lunch and dinner meal should include a small salad or steamed vegetables. It is best to use foods grown in your area and while they are in season.

Week Three – Accelerated Weight Management through Thermogenics

One of the chief drawbacks of calorie-restricted diets is their tendency to lower the body's rate of energy production. Through the thermogenic approach—the use of herbs that increase metabolism and thus burn fat faster—you do not have to abnormally restrict your caloric intake. Thermogenic herbs will help you lose weight anyway. Thermogenesis can be positively affected by green tea and the following major thermogenic herbs that are used throughout the week: kola nut, gooroo nut, yerba maté, guarana, iodine (as from fucus), white willow bark, and cayenne. Nutrients that can impact the thermogenesis process are pantothenic acid, essential fatty acids, vitamin B-6, vitamin C, ginger root, zinc, manganese, magnesium, and niacin.

Week Three Day 15

1. Do the ten-minute aromatherapy program upon awakening.
2. Thermogenic tea: have a six-ounce cup of Gingko tea with two capsules of cayenne pepper five minutes before breakfast.
3. Suggested breakfast: an eight-ounce fruit smoothie. Using pineapple, apple, or orange juices as a base, add half a banana with your choice of strawberries, blueberries, mango, peaches, apples, or pears with a pinch of nutmeg or cinnamon.
4. Have a six-ounce cup of Herba Maté ten minutes before lunch.
5. Reduce compulsive eating with Bach Remedies: ten minutes after breakfast review your emotional state and use the appropriate herbal flower remedy.
6. Suggested lunch: low-fat yogurt and half a banana.
7. Ten minutes before dinner have a six-ounce cup of ginger tea.
8. Suggested dinner: a cup of potato soup or clear vegetable broth, a small mixed green salad, and steamed cauliflower.
9. Ten minutes after dinner take one cup of Chinese Weight-loss Formula.

Week Three Day 16

1. Do the ten-minute aromatherapy program upon awakening.
2. Thermogenic tea: have a six-ounce cup of Gingko tea with two capsules of cayenne pepper five minutes before breakfast.
3. Suggested breakfast: one slice of 100 percent whole-grain toast with unsweetened fruit spread, low-fat cottage cheese, or low-fat soy cream cheese. Or, have a cup of fresh fruit salad (include apples, pears, melon, and half a banana). You may use a coffee substitute. A few available brand names include Roastarama, Pero, and Cafix.
4. Ten minutes before lunch have a six-ounce cup of Herba Maté.
5. Reduce compulsive eating with Bach Remedies: ten

minutes after breakfast review your emotional state and use the appropriate herbal flower remedy.

6. Suggested lunch: a small mixed green salad and a cup of tofu, eggless egg salad with one half toasted whole-grain pita.

7. Ten minutes before dinner have a six-ounce cup of ginger tea.

8. Suggested dinner: one cup of a steamed leafy green vegetable such as spinach, kale, collard greens, or watercress, hummus (chickpea dip), and a whole-grain pita or tortilla cut into eight pieces.

9. Ten minutes after dinner take one cup of Chinese Weight-loss Formula.

Week Three Day 17

1. Do the ten-minute aromatherapy program upon awakening.

2. Thermogenic tea: have a six-ounce cup of Gingko tea with two capsules of cayenne pepper five minutes before breakfast.

3. Suggested breakfast: one cup puffed whole-grain cereal (wheat, corn, rice, or millet) with six ounces of non-dairy soy or rice beverage. Or, have half a cantaloupe. You may use a coffee substitute. A few available brand names include Roastarama, Pero, and Cafix.

4. Ten minutes before lunch have a six-ounce cup of Herba Maté.

5. Reduce compulsive eating with Bach Remedies: ten minutes after breakfast review your emotional state and use the appropriate herbal flower remedy.

6. Suggested lunch: ten ounces Balanced Carbo-Protein Herbal Smoothie.

7. Ten minutes before dinner have a six-ounce cup of ginger tea.

8. Suggested dinner: one cup of a steamed leafy green vegetable such as spinach, kale, collard greens, or watercress, hummus (chickpea dip), and a whole-grain pita

or tortilla cut into eight pieces.

9. Ten minutes after dinner take one cup of Chinese Weight-loss Formula.

Week Three Day 18

1. Do the ten-minute aromatherapy program upon awakening.
2. Thermogenic tea: have a six-ounce cup of Gingko tea with two capsules of cayenne pepper five minutes before breakfast.
3. Suggested breakfast: an eight-ounce, high-protein smoothie. Soy or rice beverage with one teaspoon peanut butter and half a banana—add a pinch of nutmeg or cinnamon.
4. Ten minutes before lunch have a six-ounce cup of Herba Maté.
5. Reduce compulsive eating with Bach Remedies: ten minutes after breakfast review your emotional state and use the appropriate herbal flower remedy.
6. Suggested lunch: chicken-less chicken salad with alfalfa sprouts and tomato in a whole-wheat pita.
7. Ten minutes before dinner have a six-ounce cup of ginger tea.
8. Suggested dinner: one cup of a steamed green leafy vegetable such as spinach, kale, collard greens, or watercress, and black-bean dip with slices of jicima.
9. Ten minutes after dinner take one cup of Chinese Weight-loss Formula.

Week Three Day 19

1. Do the ten-minute aromatherapy program upon awakening.
2. Thermogenic tea: have a six-ounce cup of Gingko tea with two capsules of cayenne pepper five minutes before breakfast.
3. Suggested breakfast: twelve ounces of one of the Blended Drink recipes.
4. Ten minutes before lunch have a six-ounce cup of Herba Maté.
5. Reduce compulsive eating with Bach Remedies: ten

minutes after breakfast review your emotional state and use the appropriate herbal flower remedy.

6. Suggested lunch: a cup of chunky vegetable soup (broccoli, zucchini, mushrooms, carrots, water, and powdered soup mix) or clear vegetable broth, a small mixed green salad, and brown rice.

7. Ten minutes before dinner have a six-ounce cup of ginger tea.

8. Suggested dinner: one Broccoli and Garlic Stuffed Baked Potato and a small green salad, with half a whole-grain pita.

9. Ten minutes after dinner, take one cup of Chinese Weight-loss Formula.

Week Three Day 20

1. Do the ten-minute aromatherapy program upon awakening.

2. Thermogenic tea: have a six-ounce cup of Gingko tea with two capsules of cayenne pepper five minutes before breakfast.

3. Suggested breakfast: an eight-ounce fruit smoothie. Using apple juice as a base, add half a banana with your choice of strawberries, blueberries, mango, peaches, apples, or pears with a pinch of nutmeg or cinnamon.

4. Ten minutes before lunch have a six-ounce cup of Herba Maté.

5. Reduce compulsive eating with Bach Remedies: ten minutes after breakfast review your emotional state and use the appropriate herbal flower remedy.

6. Suggested lunch: low-fat yogurt and half a cup of strawberries.

7. Ten minutes before dinner have a six-ounce cup of ginger tea.

8. Suggested dinner: one cup steamed green leafy vegetable such as spinach, kale, collard greens, or watercress served with Garlic Brown Rice with soy cheese melt, a small green salad, and half a whole-grain pita.

9. Ten minutes after dinner take one cup of Chinese Weight-loss Formula.

Week Three Day 21

1. Do the ten-minute aromatherapy program upon awakening.
2. Thermogenic tea: have a six-ounce cup of Gingko tea with two capsules of cayenne pepper five minutes before breakfast.
3. Suggested breakfast: an eight-ounce fruit smoothie. Using pineapple, orange, or apple juice as a base, add half a banana with your choice of strawberries, blueberries, mango, peaches, apples, or pears with a pinch of nutmeg or cinnamon.
4. Ten minutes before lunch have a six-ounce cup of Herba Maté.
5. Reduce compulsive eating with Bach Remedies: ten minutes after breakfast review your emotional state and use the appropriate herbal flower remedy.
6. Suggested lunch: low-fat yogurt and half a cup of peach and plum combination.
7. Ten minutes before dinner have a six-ounce cup of ginger tea.
8. Suggested dinner: one cup of a steamed green leafy vegetable such as spinach, kale, collard greens, or watercress, white bean dip, and whole-grain pita or tortilla cut into eight pieces.
9. Ten minutes after dinner take one cup of Chinese Weight-loss Formula.

Tips for Week Three:

- Many individuals who are overweight find that they need a little help to "jump start" their ability to burn fat. Certain herbs can promote thermogenesis, which occurs in brown adipose tissue and reverses the body's tendency to store fat by increasing the production of heat-energy, which burns calories.

- Top pizza with vegetables and a sprinkling of cheese.
- Try cheeses naturally lower in fat, such as feta and part-skim mozzarella. Also try soy-based cheeses or the reduced-fat cheeses now on the market.

Week Four—Stabilized Weight Management

This program will help support and maintain a steady weight loss until you reach your desired weight.

Week Four Day 22

1. Five minutes before breakfast have a six-ounce cup of green tea.
2. Suggested breakfast: Spanish-style half tofu scramble with sautéed peppers, onions, and tomatoes (sautéed in non-fat spray). You may use a coffee substitute. A few available brand names include Roastarama, Pero, and Cafix.
3. Ten minutes after breakfast take one 750 mg tablet of Hydroxycitric (HCA, an herbal extract).
4. Reduce compulsive eating with Bach Remedies: ten minutes after breakfast review your emotional state and use the appropriate herbal flower remedy.
5. Eat a snack within two hours of breakfast. You want to use foods that will cause a slow release of sugar, which evens out the distribution of glucose. One hundred percent whole-wheat toast with sugar-free fruit spread or a rice cake with cottage cheese is a good choice.
6. Suggested lunch: ten ounces Balanced Carbo-Protein Herbal Smoothie.
7. Have a snack of celery sticks or apple slices and cottage cheese. These can be alternated with whole fruit such as peaches, plums, and mangoes. Eat one or two snacks in the afternoon, spaced no farther than three hours apart. This "snack spacing" will help support creation of a balance in your blood sugar while increasing your metabolism.

8. Have a cup of the Weight-Reducing Formula consisting of:
   Dandelion root and leaves (7 parts)
   Peppermint leaves (7 parts)
   Alder buckthorn bark (15 parts)
9. Remember: eat dinner by no later than 8 P.M., if possible. Try my Spicy Portobello-Sage Stuffing (see recipe) and a small green salad with thermogenic dressing.
10. Ten minutes after dinner take one cup of alfalfa-leaf tea.

Week Four Day 23

1. Five minutes before breakfast have a six-ounce cup of green tea.
2. Suggested breakfast should consist of a carbohydrate, or whole-grain cereal for quick energy, and a protein, such as a soy shake, for a more lasting boost.
3. Ten minutes after breakfast take one 750 mg tablet of Hydroxycitric (HCA, an herbal extract).
4. Reduce compulsive eating with Bach Remedies: ten minutes after breakfast review your emotional state and use the appropriate herbal flower remedy.
5. Eat a snack within two hours of breakfast. You want to use foods that will cause a slow release of sugar, which evens out the distribution of glucose. One hundred percent whole-wheat toast with sugar-free fruit spread or a rice cake with cottage cheese is a good choice.
6. Suggested lunch: mixed herb/vegetable soup, a baked cauliflower with herbal seasonings with a serving of an herbed whole-grain dish, such as rice, kasha, or polenta.
7. Have a snack of celery sticks or apple slices and cottage cheese. These can be alternated with whole fruit such as peaches, plums, and mangoes. Eat one or two snacks in the afternoon, spaced no further than three hours apart. This "snack spacing" will help support creation of a balance in your blood sugar while increasing your metabolism.

8. Have a cup of the Weight-Reducing Formula consisting of:
   Dandelion root and leaves (7 parts)
   Peppermint leaves (7 parts)
   Alder buckthorn bark (15 parts)
9. Remember: eat dinner by no later than 8 P.M., if possible. Try a cup of soup and Curry Baked Tofu.
10. Ten minutes after dinner take one cup of alfalfa-leaf tea.

Week Four Day 24

1. Five minutes before breakfast have a six-ounce cup of green tea.
2. Suggested breakfast: Spanish-style half tofu scramble with sautéed peppers, onions, and tomatoes (sautéed in non-fat spray). You may use a coffee substitute. A few available brand names include Roastarama, Pero, and Cafix.
3. Ten minutes after breakfast take one 750 mg tablet of Hydroxycitric (HCA, an herbal extract).
4. Reduce compulsive eating with Bach Remedies: ten minutes after breakfast review your emotional state and use the appropriate herbal flower remedy.
5. Eat a snack within two hours of breakfast. You want to use foods that will cause a slow release of sugar, which evens out the distribution of glucose. One hundred percent whole-wheat toast with sugar-free fruit spread or a rice cake with cottage cheese is a good choice.
6. Suggested lunch: ten ounces Balanced Carbo-Protein Herbal Smoothie or instead have mixed herb/vegetable soup, a baked cauliflower with herbal seasonings with a serving of an herbed whole-grain dish such as rice, kasha, or polenta.
7. Have a snack of celery sticks or apple slices and cottage cheese. These can be alternated with whole fruit such as peaches, plums, and mangoes. Eat one or two snacks in the afternoon, spaced no further than three hours apart. This "snack spacing" will help support creation of a balance in

your blood sugar while increasing your metabolism.

8. Have a cup of the Weight-Reducing Formula consisting of:
   Dandelion root and leaves (7 parts)
   Peppermint leaves (7 parts)
   Alder buckthorn bark (15 parts)
9. Try my Herbed Tofu Pilaf (see recipe) and a small salad with thermogenic dressing.
10. Ten minutes after dinner take one cup of alfalfa-leaf tea.

Week Four Day 25

1. Five minutes before breakfast have a six-ounce cup of green tea.
2. Suggested breakfast: one cup of fresh fruit salad (include apples, pears, melon, and half a banana). Or, have half a cantaloupe. You may use a coffee substitute. A few available brand names include Roastarama, Pero, and Cafix.
3. Ten minutes after breakfast take one 750 mg tablet of Hydroxycitric (HCA, an herbal extract).
4. Reduce compulsive eating with Bach Remedies: ten minutes after breakfast review your emotional state and use the appropriate herbal flower remedy.
5. Eat a snack within two hours of breakfast. You want to use foods that will cause a slow release of sugar, which evens out the distribution of glucose. One hundred percent whole-wheat toast with sugar-free fruit spread or a rice cake with cottage cheese is a good choice.
6. Suggested lunch: ten ounces Balanced Carbo-Protein Herbal Smoothie or instead have mixed herb/vegetable soup, a baked cauliflower with herbal seasonings with a serving of an herbed whole-grain dish such as rice, kasha, or polenta.
7. Have a snack of celery sticks or apple slices and cottage cheese. These can be alternated with whole fruit such as peaches, plums, and mangoes. Eat one or two snacks in the afternoon, spaced no further than three hours apart. This

"snack spacing" will help support creation of a balance in your blood sugar while increasing your metabolism.

8. Have a cup of the Weight-Reducing Formula consisting of:
   Dandelion root and leaves (7 parts)
   Peppermint leaves (7 parts)
   Alder buckthorn bark (15 parts)

9. Suggested dinner: one cup of any steamed vegetable or combination of vegetables (broccoli, zucchini, kale, carrots, and yellow squash are good choices), a cup of Mock-Chicken Salad, and half a toasted pita.

10. Ten minutes after dinner take one cup of alfalfa-leaf tea.

Week Four Day 26

1. Five minutes before breakfast have a six-ounce cup of green tea.

2. Suggested breakfast: an eight-ounce fruit smoothie. Using pineapple, apple, or orange juice as a base, add half a banana with your choice of strawberries, blueberries, mango, peaches, apples, or pears with a pinch of nutmeg or cinnamon.

3. Ten minutes after breakfast take one 750 mg tablet of Hydroxycitric (HCA, an herbal extract).

4. Reduce compulsive eating with Bach Remedies: ten minutes after breakfast review your emotional state and use the appropriate herbal flower remedy.

5. Eat a snack within two hours of breakfast. You want to use foods that will cause a slow release of sugar, which evens out the distribution of glucose. One hundred percent whole-wheat toast with sugar-free fruit spread or a rice cake with cottage cheese is a good choice.

6. Suggested lunch: ten ounces Balanced Carbo-Protein Herbal Smoothie or instead have mixed herb/vegetable soup, a baked cauliflower with herbal seasonings with a serving of an herbed whole-grain dish such as rice, kasha, or polenta.

7. Have a snack of celery sticks or apple slices and cottage cheese. These can be alternated with whole fruit such as peaches, plums, and mangoes. Eat one or two snacks in the afternoon, spaced no further than three hours apart. This "snack spacing" will help support creation of a balance in your blood sugar while increasing your metabolism.

8. Have a cup of the Weight-Reducing Formula consisting of:
   Dandelion root and leaves (7 parts)
   Peppermint leaves (7 parts)
   Alder buckthorn bark (15 parts)

9. Suggested dinner: Mock Lasagna (see recipe at back of book) and a small green salad.

10. Ten minutes after dinner take one cup of alfalfa-leaf tea.

Week Four Day 27

1. Five minutes before breakfast have a six-ounce cup of green tea.

2. Suggested breakfast: an eight-ounce, high-protein smoothie: soy or rice beverage, one teaspoon peanut butter, and one teaspoon of coffee substitute.

3. Ten minutes after breakfast take one 750 mg tablet of Hydroxycitric (HCA, an herbal extract).

4. Reduce compulsive eating with Bach Remedies: ten minutes after breakfast review your emotional state and use the appropriate herbal flower remedy.

5. Eat a snack within two hours of breakfast. You want to use foods that will cause a slow release of sugar, which evens out the distribution of glucose. One hundred percent whole-wheat toast with sugar-free fruit spread or a rice cake with cottage cheese is a good choice.

6. Suggested lunch: ten ounces Balanced Carbo-Protein Herbal Smoothie or instead have mixed herb/vegetable soup, a baked cauliflower with herbal seasonings with a serving of an herbed whole-grain dish such as rice, kasha, or polenta.

7. Have a snack of celery sticks or apple slices and cottage cheese. These can be alternated with whole fruit such as peaches, plums, and mangoes. Eat one or two snacks in the afternoon, spaced no further than three hours apart. This "snack spacing" will help support creation of a balance in your blood sugar while increasing your metabolism.

8. Have a cup of the Weight-Reducing Formula consisting of:
   Dandelion root and leaves (7 parts)
   Peppermint leaves (7 parts)
   Alder buckthorn bark (15 parts)

9. Suggested dinner: Poblano Chilies with Black Beans and Soy Cheese and a small green salad.

10. Ten minutes after dinner take one cup of alfalfa-leaf tea.

Week Four Day 28

1. Five minutes before breakfast have a six-ounce cup of green tea.

2. Suggested breakfast should consist of a carbohydrate, or whole-grain cereal for quick energy, and a protein, such as a soy shake, for a more lasting boost.

3. Ten minutes after breakfast take one 750 mg tablet of Hydroxycitric (HCA, an herbal extract).

4. Reduce compulsive eating with Bach Remedies: ten minutes after breakfast review your emotional state and use the appropriate herbal flower remedy.

5. Eat a snack within two hours of breakfast. You want to use foods that will cause a slow release of sugar, which evens out the distribution of glucose. One hundred percent whole-wheat toast with sugar-free fruit spread or a rice cake with cottage cheese is a good choice.

6. Suggested lunch: ten ounces Balanced Carbo-Protein Herbal Smoothie or instead have mixed herb/vegetable soup, a baked cauliflower with herbal seasonings with a serving of an herbed whole-grain dish such as rice, kasha, or polenta.

7. Have a snack of celery sticks or apple slices and cottage cheese. These can be alternated with whole fruit such as peaches, plums, and mangoes. Eat one or two snacks in the afternoon, spaced no further than three hours apart. This "snack spacing" will help support creation of a balance in your blood sugar while increasing your metabolism.

8. Have a cup of the Weight-Reducing Formula consisting of:
   Dandelion root and leaves (7 parts)
   Peppermint leaves (7 parts)
   Alder buckthorn bark (15 parts)

9. Pick any dinner choice and finish the meal no later than 8 P.M., if possible. As with lunch, focus on soup, protein (low-fat cheese, beans, tofu, soy milk, or, if you are not a vegetarian, lean skinless chicken or fish), and vegetables, along with a cup of pasta with one of the herbed sauces listed in the book.

10. Ten minutes after dinner take one cup of alfalfa-leaf tea.

Maintenance Program Day 29

1. Five minutes before breakfast have a six-ounce cup of green tea.

2. Suggested breakfast should consist of a carbohydrate, or whole-grain cereal for quick energy, and a protein, such as a soy shake, for a more lasting boost.

3. Ten minutes after breakfast, take one 750 mg tablet of Hydroxycitric (HCA, an herbal extract).

4. Reduce compulsive eating with Bach Remedies: ten minutes after breakfast review your emotional state and use the appropriate herbal flower remedy.

5. Eat a snack within two hours of breakfast. You want to use foods that will cause a slow release of sugar, which evens out the distribution of glucose. One hundred percent whole-wheat toast with sugar-free fruit spread or a rice cake with cottage cheese is a good choice.

6. Suggested lunch: ten ounces Balanced Carbo-Protein Herbal Smoothie or instead have mixed herb/vegetable soup, a baked cauliflower with herbal seasonings with a serving of an herbed whole-grain dish such as rice, kasha, or polenta.

7. Have a snack of celery sticks or apple slices and cottage cheese. These can be alternated with whole fruit such as peaches, plums, and mangoes. Eat one or two snacks in the afternoon, spaced no further than three hours apart. This "snack spacing" will help support creation of a balance in your blood sugar while increasing your metabolism.

8. Have a cup of the Weight-Reducing Formula consisting of:
   Dandelion root and leaves (7 parts)
   Peppermint leaves (7 parts)
   Alder buckthorn bark (15 parts)

9. Suggested dinner: one cup of a steamed green leafy vegetable such as spinach, kale, collard greens, or watercress, black-bean humus and whole-grain pita bread or tortilla cut into eight pieces.

10. Ten minutes after dinner take one cup of alfalfa-leaf tea.

Maintenance Program Day 30

1. Five minutes before breakfast have a six-ounce cup of green tea.

2. Suggested breakfast should consist of a carbohydrate, or whole-grain cereal for quick energy, and a protein, such as a soy shake, for a more lasting boost.

3. Ten minutes after breakfast, take one 750 mg tablet of Hydroxycitric (HCA, an herbal extract).

4. Reduce compulsive eating with Bach Remedies: ten minutes after breakfast review your emotional state and use the appropriate herbal flower remedy.

5. Eat a snack within two hours of breakfast. You want to use foods that will cause a slow release of sugar, which

evens out the distribution of glucose. One hundred percent whole-wheat toast with sugar-free fruit spread or a rice cake with cottage cheese is a good choice.

6. Suggested lunch: ten ounces Balanced Carbo-Protein Herbal Smoothie or instead have mixed herb/vegetable soup, a baked cauliflower with herbal seasonings with a serving of an herbed whole-grain dish such as rice, kasha, or polenta.

7. Have a snack of celery sticks or apple slices and cottage cheese. These can be alternated with whole fruit such as peaches, plums, and mangoes. Eat one or two snacks in the afternoon, spaced no further than three hours apart. This "snack spacing" will help support creation of a balance in your blood sugar while increasing your metabolism.

8. Have a cup of the Weight-Reducing Formula consisting of:
   Dandelion root and leaves (7 parts)
   Peppermint leaves (7 parts)
   Alder buckthorn bark (15 parts)

9. Suggested dinner: a grilled vegetable sandwich. Grill or roast zucchini and peppers and serve them on whole-grain bread with mustard or low-fat salad dressing. Add lettuce, tomato, and pickles.

10. Ten minutes after dinner take one cup of alfalfa-leaf tea.

Tips for Week Four

• Reduce or replace the creams used for thickening. Try low-fat or non-fat yogurt in recipes that call for sweet or sour cream. Use arrowroot powder, potatoes, or rice flour to thicken soups.

• Add herbs, salt, pepper, Stevia as a sweetener, lemon, cider vinegar, natural tamari soy sauce, mustard, and ketchup (homemade or from a natural foods store) to your foods if you like.

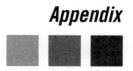
List of Recipes

If you love to cook but are trying to stay on your herbal weight-loss program, these recipes are for you. With a few exceptions, they take some preparation time but are rich in flavor, texture, good nutrition, and are low in fat and calories. All recipes are designed to produce three to four low-fat, high-fiber, herb-rich portions so they can be served in a family setting or with friends. If you are eating alone the remaining servings can be refrigerated for three to four days or frozen.

Herbal Soup Recipes

Most herbal soup recipes take a total of fifteen to thirty minutes of preparation and cooking time. These recipes are designed to create three to four servings. They can be eaten as a six-ounce serving either at lunch or dinner.

Hearty Split Pea Soup
Ingredients:
> *1-½ cups split peas*
> *½ lb. low-fat tofu (meatless) hot dogs*
> *1 bay leaf*
> *3 tsp.*
> *1 large natural vegetable bouillon cube or powder*
> *1 clove garlic, smashed and chopped*
> *1 medium yellow onion, chopped*

1 large carrot, chopped
2 stalks celery, chopped
½ red bell pepper, chopped
¼ cup plus 1 Tbsp. whole-wheat flour
½ cup rice or soy milk
Whole-grain sourdough bread
Freshly ground black pepper to taste
⅛ tsp. cayenne
2 Tbsp. fresh parsley, chopped fine
¾ cup plain non-fat yogurt, stirred smooth

Preparation Instructions:

Wash and sort split peas in colander. Place tofu hot dogs, split peas, and all but the last seven ingredients in large iron or stainless steel-bottomed saucepan. Bring to a boil over high heat. Reduce heat to low, cover, and cook twenty minutes. Shake flour and soy or rice milk vigorously in container with tight-fitting lid. Shake until all lumps have disappeared. Stir gradually into boiling mixture. Wrap bread in foil and place in warm oven.

Reduce heat under soup to low. Cook ten minutes. Stir often.

Add black pepper, cayenne, and parsley. Cook five minutes. Stir in yogurt just prior to serving. Remove from heat. Serve with warm sourdough bread.

Smooth Tomato Soup

Ingredients:

4 tomatoes, peeled and finely chopped
3 cups vegetable stock (This can be made with natural
  vegetable stock cube, crumbled or powder)
1 onion, minced
2 whole cloves
1 tsp. dried basil, or 1 Tbsp. fresh basil, chopped
1-½ Tbsp. non-fat powdered butter replacement
1-½ Tbsp. whole-grain flour
1 tsp. honey
2 cups plain rice or soy milk, hot

Preparation Instructions:
Combine first five ingredients in a heavy iron or stainless steel saucepan over low heat. Cover and simmer thirty minutes. Remove from heat. Strain mixture through a fine sieve. Stir in salt and pepper to taste. Using a wooden spoon, combine powdered butter substitute and flour in a small bowl. Add flour paste and honey to tomato mixture. Whisk over medium heat until mixture thickens slightly. Remove tomato mixture from heat. Stir hot rice or soy milk very slowly into tomato mixture so mixture will not curdle. Return tomato soup to medium low heat until very hot but not boiling.

Vegetable and Barley Soup
Ingredients:
- ⅓ cup plus 3 Tbsp. pearl barley
- 3-¼ cups water
- 1 medium onion, chopped
- 1 clove garlic, crushed
- 1 stick celery, chopped
- 2 medium carrots, chopped
- 1 medium potato, chopped
- 1 lb. canned, crushed tomatoes
- 1 large natural vegetable stock cube, crumbled (or powder)
- 2-¾ Tbsp. fresh parsley, chopped

Preparation Instructions:
Soak barley in the water overnight. Use nonstick lecithin/vegetable spray in a heavy saucepan over medium heat and cook next five ingredients about three minutes, stirring until onion is soft. Add remaining ingredients, except parsley. Add undrained barley and water mixture. Bring to a boil over high heat. Reduce heat, cover, and simmer about fifteen minutes or until vegetables are tender. Stir in the parsley just before serving.

Carrot Soup with Spinach

Ingredients:

1 lb. carrots, scrubbed

1 small parsnip, peeled and chopped

1 small onion, peeled and quartered

1 celery rib, cut into 2-inch pieces

3 cups vegetable stock (made with vegetable stock cube,
     crumbled, or powder)

¼ tsp. nutmeg

¼ lb. spinach leaves, rinsed and tough stems discarded

1 cup whole-grain croutons

Salt and pepper to taste

Preparation Instructions:

Combine first five ingredients and cook over high heat in a heavy skillet, or using nonstick lecithin/vegetable spray on a stainless steel pan. Cover and bring vegetable stock to a boil. Reduce heat to low and simmer thirty minutes. Transfer vegetables to a food processor or blender. Add a small amount of vegetable liquid and pureed vegetables. Return puree to saucepan with stock. Add nutmeg and salt and pepper to taste. Place spinach in a food processor or blender. Add one cup of soup to spinach and puree. Stir spinach puree into soup and serve hot with croutons.

Carrot Yam Soup

Ingredients:

1 pound sliced carrots (do not peel if organic)

1 small red onion, chopped

Nonstick vegetable spray

3 cups vegetable broth

Salt and pepper to taste

1 cup steamed yams pureed

Preparation Instructions:

In a large saucepan, combine carrots and onions. Saute about two minutes with nonstick vegetable spray. Add broth. Heat over medium heat until it boils, then reduce the heat and simmer about twenty minutes or until carrots are very tender. Stir in the yams. Place the mixture in a blender or food processor. Process until the soup is smooth and thickened. Serve immediately.

Seitan, Corn, and Tomato Chowder
Ingredients:
> 1-½ lbs. Seitan Nuggets
> 2 cups water
> ½ medium onion, chopped
> ½ tsp. natural vegetable stock cube, crumbled, or powder
> ½ lb. canned creamed corn
> ½ lb. canned whole tomatoes, drained and cut up
> ½ tsp. lemon juice

Preparation Instructions:
Bring first four ingredients to a boil in a large pot over high heat. Simmer twenty minutes. Combine seitan, vegetable broth, and remaining ingredients in a stainless steel pot. Add salt and pepper to taste.

Herb and Vegetable Salad Recipes

Most salad recipes take a total of ten to twenty minutes of preparation time. These recipes are designed to create three to four servings. Have a small salad at the beginning of each lunch and dinner meal. You can also have them at snack time.

Japanese Cabbage Salad
Ingredients:
> 1 grated carrot
> 1 cup chopped cucumber
> 1 tsp. sesame seeds
> ¼ cup cubed, firm tofu
> 1 medium tomato, sliced
> 1 cup grated cabbage

Preparation Instructions:
Combine the ingredients and add lemon juice, a natural food brand dressing, or low-fat salad dressing.

Mock-Chicken Salad
Ingredients:

> 2 or 3 cups TVP (Textured Vegetable Protein)
> ½ cup sliced fresh mushrooms
> ½ cup thinly sliced celery
> 2 Tbsp. chopped Vidalia onion
> ½ cup grated carrots
> ⅛ cup chopped red bell peppers
> ⅛ cup chopped yellow bell peppers
> 2 Tbsp. of eggless, low-fat, tofu-based mayonnaise
>   (available at your health-food store)

Preparation Instructions:
Combine the TVP, mushrooms, celery, green onion, carrots, and red bell peppers. Add tofu-based mayonnaise and toss until well mixed. Arrange on romaine and Boston lettuce leaves on a large salad plate or on individual plates. Garnish with yellow bell pepper.

Tempeh Salad
Ingredients:

> ½ cup cooked brown rice, chilled
> ¼ cup thinly sliced celery
> 2 Tbsp. thinly sliced green onions with tops
> ⅛ cup sliced radishes
> ¾ cup fresh bean sprouts, drained
> 1-½ cups thinly slivered Tempeh
> ⅛ cup chopped red bell peppers
> ⅛ cup almonds
> 1 tsp. raw sesame seeds
> ¾ Tbsp. low sodium soy sauce
> 1-½ Tbsp. apple cider vinegar
> 2 Tbsp. almond or olive oil

1 cup romaine or Boston lettuce
½ fresh nectarine or peach slices

Preparation Instructions:
In a large bowl combine rice, celery, onions, radishes, bean sprouts, Tempeh, and ⅛ cup of the almonds. Measure sesame seed, soy sauce, vinegar, and oil into small jar. Cover and shake well. Pour over rice mixture and toss thoroughly. Spoon into lettuce-lined bowl; chill. To serve, garnish with nectarine slices.

Mixed Vegetable Salad

Ingredients:
1 grated carrot
1 cup chopped cucumber
1 medium tomato, sliced
1 cup romaine lettuce

Preparation Instructions:
Combine the ingredients and add lemon juice or a natural food brand or low-fat salad dressing.

Dips and Sauces

Creamy Garlic Dip with Vegetables

Ingredients:
2 cups plain non-fat yogurt
1-½ Tbsp. chopped fresh garlic
¼ tsp. powdered onion soup mix
½ tsp. grated organic lemon peel
½ tsp. fresh lemon juice
¼ tsp. salt
¼ tsp. pepper
A pinch cayenne pepper
1-½ kirby cucumbers, thinly sliced
8 oz. cherry tomatoes

Preparation Instructions:
Place strainer over four-cup measuring cup. Line strainer with paper towel. Add yogurt to strainer; chill until yogurt is thick

(about one cup liquid will drain from yogurt), at least two hours or overnight. Turn yogurt out into medium bowl; discard paper towel and drained liquid. To make the non-fat yogurt closer in consistency to sour cream, add chopped fresh garlic and onion soup powder, lemon peel, lemon juice, salt, pepper, and cayenne to yogurt and stir to blend. Cover and refrigerate to develop flavors, at least two hours and up to six hours. Place bowl with dip on platter. Surround with sliced cucumbers and cherry tomatoes and serve. Makes four servings (about 1¼ cups of dip).

Based on a recipe in *Bon Appétit,* June 1997.

Non-fat Tomato Sauce
Ingredients:

>   *1 Tbsp. olive oil*
>   *Nonstick vegetable spray*
>   *1 Tbsp. finely minced garlic*
>   *2 cups crushed tomatoes*
>   *1 tsp. crumbled oregano*
>   *½ tsp. dried rosemary*
>   *Salt to taste, if desired*
>   *Freshly ground pepper to taste*
>   *2 Tbsp. finely chopped fresh basil*

Preparation Instructions:

Spray the pan with nonstick vegetable spray and heat the oil. Add the garlic and cook briefly, stirring. Add the tomatoes, oregano, rosemary, salt, and pepper. Bring to a boil and cook, stirring occasionally, about fifteen minutes. Stir in the basil and serve hot. Yields about one and one-half cups.

Cucumber Garlic Dressing
Ingredients:

>   *1 cup cucumbers*
>   *¼ cup chopped onion*
>   *1 clove garlic*
>   *¼ cup red wine vinegar*

½ cup chopped basil
Chopped parsley to taste

Preparation Instructions:

Blend ingredients together in a food processor or blender. Use to taste on salad.

Ginger Tahini

Ingredients:

2 cups water
2 cups hulled sesame seeds or sesame tahini
    (pour off the oil from the tahini before blending)
¼ cup lemon juice
2 cloves garlic
¼ cup tamari
2 Tbsp. grated ginger

Preparation Instructions:

Blend ingredients together in a food processor or blender. Use to taste on salad.

Dill Mustard

Ingredients:

2 Tbsp. dijon mustard
¼ cup apple-cider vinegar
1 clove garlic
½ cup water
Fresh parsley and dill
A dash cayenne pepper

Preparation Instructions:

Blend ingredients together in a food processor or blender. Use to taste on salad.

Entrée Recipes

Entrées can be used as main dishes at lunch or dinner. They are offered as a source of variety during your meals. Remember to exercise portion control and use in combination with soups and simple salads. Most of the entrée recipes presented here take a total of fifteen to forty-five minutes of preparation and cooking time. These recipes are designed to create three to four servings. They can be eaten as a six-ounce serving either at lunch or dinner.

Couscous-Stuffed Tomatoes with Raisins and Herbs

Ingredients:

    2-½ lb. tomatoes
    ⅛ cup raisins
    About ¾ cup vegetable broth
    ½ Tbsp. olive oil
    ½ cup couscous
    1 oz. finely chopped scallion
    ½ Tbsp. minced fresh dill
    ½ Tbsp. minced fresh mint leaves
    1 Tbsp. fresh lemon juice
    Salt and pepper to taste

Preparation Instructions:

Halve each tomato horizontally, scoop out, and discard the seeds. With a grapefruit knife, scoop out the pulp, reserving it and leaving ⅓-inch-thick shells. Sprinkle the insides of the tomatoes with salt and invert the tomato shells onto a rack to drain for thirty minutes. In a small saucepan, combine the raisins with half a cup of the broth and simmer them for five minutes. Drain the raisins in a sieve set over a two-cup measure. Add enough of the remaining broth to measure ¾ cups, and transfer the broth to the pan. Add half a tablespoon of the oil to the broth and bring the mixture to a boil. Stir in the couscous and let it stand, covered, off the heat for five minutes. Stir the couscous with a fork, breaking up any lumps, and toss it in a bowl with the currants, the reserved tomato pulp, chopped, the remaining one tablespoon of oil, the scallion, the dill, the mint, the lemon juice, and salt and pepper to taste. Divide the couscous mixture among the tomato shells, mounding it. Spray the baking dish with nonstick lecithin/vegetable spray. Arrange the stuffed tomatoes in a baking dish just large enough to hold them, and bake them, covered, in a pre-heated 325°F oven for ten minutes. Serve the stuffed tomatoes warm or at room temperature.

Baked Herbed Tomatoes

Ingredients:

> 2 tomatoes, halved horizontally and seeded
> 1 cup fine whole-grain bread crumbs
>   (available in health-food stores)
> ¼ cup finely chopped onion
> ½ tsp. minced garlic
> ½ cup finely chopped fresh basil leaves
> ¼ tsp. dried thyme, crumbled
> 2 tsp. extra-virgin olive oil
> Salt and pepper to taste

Preparation Instructions:

Sprinkle the insides of the tomatoes with salt, arrange the tomato halves, cut side down, on layers of paper towels, and let them drain for one hour. In a bowl stir together the bread crumbs, the onion, the garlic, the basil, the thyme, and salt and pepper to taste and stir in the oil. Arrange the tomato halves, cut side up, in a shallow baking pan, and divide the bread crumb mixture among them. The tomatoes may be prepared up to this point four hours in advance and kept at room temperature. Bake the tomatoes in the upper third of a preheated 450°F oven for ten minutes or until the topping is golden. Do not overcook the tomatoes or they will lose their shape.

Garlic Onion and Sage Stuffing

Ingredients:

> 2-½ Tbsp. extra-virgin olive oil
> 1-½ small onions, finely chopped
> 1-½ celery stalks, diced
> 2-½ garlic cloves, chopped
> 18-oz. whole-grain bread

4 Tbsp. rubbed or ground dried sage
Salt to taste (a little less than ½ tsp.)
¾ tsp. dried oregano, crumbled
¾ tsp. dried thyme, crumbled
¾ tsp. pepper
¾ tsp. Italian seasoning
Egg replacement (equivalent to 2½ eggs)
¾ cup vegetable broth

Preparation Instructions:

Place oil in heavy, large skillet over medium heat. Add onions, celery, and garlic and sauté until soft, about eight minutes. Place bread in food processor and combine with sage, salt, oregano, thyme, pepper, and Italian seasoning in large bowl. Stir in onion mixture and egg replacer. Add broth and mix well.

Curried Rice

Ingredients:

1 cup brown rice
3 cups spring or distilled water
½ tsp. salt
½ clove garlic, slivered
¼ cup chopped onion
¼ cup chopped green pepper
¹⁄₁₆ cup sesame tahini
⅛ tsp. curry powder

Preparation Instructions:

Wash rice, then add to three cups boiling, salted water. Bring to a boil again, let boil for a minute, then reduce heat and simmer, covered, about one hour. Meanwhile, place frying pan on medium heat and spray with nonstick vegetable spray. When the pan is hot, add onion and garlic and stir for a minute or two. Add green pepper, curry, and a pinch of salt and stir for another few minutes. Add one cup water, reduce heat, and simmer with lid ajar for ten minutes or so until liquid is half gone. Combine curry mixture with rice about fifteen minutes before rice is done, mixing gently to keep rice fluffy (long-grain rice tends to cook fluffier than short or medium grain). Cook together without stirring until done, mix once lightly, and serve.

Italian Sloppy Joes
Ingredients:
  ¼ cup of dry TVP (Textured Vegetable Protein)
  4–7 oz. of spring or distilled water
  ½ lb. crushed tomatoes
  2 Tbsp. honey
  1 whole-grain burger roll
  Nonstick spray
  A pinch of oregano
  1 clove fresh, chopped garlic
  1½ small onions

Preparation Instructions:
Heat the water just until it is warm and add the TVP until it is soft. Strain off the excess water. Sauté the chopped onions and garlic in a frying pan coated with nonstick spray. Stir in crushed tomatoes. Season with salt and pepper to taste. Cook two minutes or until heated through. Spoon onto rolls.

Curry Baked Tofu
Ingredients
  1-¾ lbs. of cubed tofu
  ⅔ cup dairy low-fat yogurt (or soy or seed yogurt)
  ⅛ tsp. paprika
  1/16 tsp. curry powder
  ½ tsp. onion powder
  1 cup diced, roasted almonds

Preparation Instructions:
Mix together low-fat yogurt, onion powder, paprika, and curry powder. Dip tofu into yogurt-curry mixture. Roll tofu pieces in almonds and arrange on flat baking pan. Bake in 350°F oven for about twenty-five minutes.

Hot Greens
Ingredients
> ¼ cup vegetable broth
>
> 1 tsp. olive oil
>
> 2 cloves of garlic
>
> ¼ cup chopped onion
>
> 1 Tbsp. prepared mustard
>
> 2 Tbsp. prepared horseradish
>
> 6 cups shredded greens (collard, kale, mustard, etc.)
>
> ¼ cup soy "sour cream" (optional)

Preparation Instructions:
Briefly sauté garlic and onion over low heat in broth and olive oil. Stir in mustard, horseradish, and raw, shredded greens. Cover and cook over low heat until wilted. Stir occasionally to prevent burning. Makes a great accompaniment for veggie burgers or cooked beans.

Stuffed Totillas with Cottage Cheese, Green Bell Peppers, and Tomato Sauce
Ingredients for the Filling:
> 1 small green bell pepper, minced
>
> ⅛ cup olive oil
>
> ½ garlic clove, minced
>
> 8 oz. low-fat cottage cheese
>
> ¼ cup freshly grated Parmesan
>
> ¾ cup tomato sauce

Ingredients for the Tomato Sauce:
> 7- to 8-ounces canned plum tomatoes including the juice
>
> ¼ tsp. sea salt, or to taste
>
> ¼ tsp. honey or sucanet
>
> 1 Tbsp. tomato paste
>
> ¼ tsp. dried basil, crumbled
>
> A pinch of cayenne, or to taste
>
> ⅓ cup peeled, seeded, and diced fresh tomatoes

Ingredients for the Jacket:
> 1 whole-grain tortilla or Chapatti

⅓ cup minced fresh parsley leaves or a mixture of other
minced fresh herbs such as chives, coriander, or tarragon
Melted, unsalted butter for brushing the pan

Preparation Instructions:

Cook the bell pepper over moderately low heat in the oil in a heavy nonstick skillet or using nonstick lecithin/vegetable spray on a stainless steel pan. Stir until the pepper is softened, add the garlic, and cook the mixture, stirring, for one minute. In a bowl stir together the bell pepper mixture, the cottage cheese, and ¼ cup of the Parmesan with sea salt and white pepper to taste, letting the filling cool. Spread about two tablespoons of the filling on each tortilla, and roll up jelly roll fashion. Arrange the tortilla, seam sides down, in a shallow baking dish just large enough to hold them in one layer, sprayed with not-stick vegetable spray. Sprinkle them with the remaining Parmesan. Bake the tortillas in the middle of a preheated 300°F oven for twenty minutes and serve them with the sauce.

Preparing Tomato Sauce:

Force the canned tomatoes with the juice through a food mill into a saucepan. Stir in the salt, honey, tomato paste, basil, and cayenne. Bring the mixture to a boil, and simmer, stirring, for twenty minutes. Add the fresh tomatoes and cook the mixture for five minutes. Serve the sauce warm. Makes a little less than ¾ cup. Makes four stuffed tortillas, serving two to three.

Pizza-Style, Herb-Stuffed Potato

Ingredients:

4 large baking potatoes
2 cups TVP (Textured Vegetable Protein)
⅓ cup onion, finely chopped
⅓ cup green bell pepper, seeded and chopped
¼ cup mushrooms, chopped
2 tsp. parsley flakes
2 tsp. Italian herb seasoning
1 tsp. garlic powder

1 tsp. oregano
½ cup non-fat yogurt
1 cup shredded part-skim mozzarella cheese
½ cup crushed tomatoes
12 black olives (optional), sliced
2 Tbsp. grated Parmesan cheese

Preparation Instructions:

Preheat oven to 400°F. Pierce potatoes with a fork or sharp knife and microwave on high for ten to twelve minutes, or place in oven for twenty minutes. Cool slightly. Heat a heavy nonstick skillet over medium-high heat or use nonstick lecithin/vegetable spray on a stainless steel pan. Boil two cups of water and place TVP in it. Let cook for five minutes. Pour off excess water. Stir in the next three ingredients and cook two minutes. Stir in parsley, Italian seasoning, and garlic powder. Split each potato lengthwise and scoop out pulp with a soup spoon into a bowl. Combine yogurt and salt and pepper to taste with pulp and mix well. Stir in ⅔ cup part-skim mozzarella and TVP mixture. Mix thoroughly. Stuff potato shells with mixture. Heat crushed tomatoes. Add garlic powder, onion powder, oregano, and salt to taste. Top each potato with sauce, remaining mozzarella, olives, and Parmesan. Bake twenty minutes or until bubbly.

Vegetable Nachos

Ingredients:

64 baked (no oil) whole-corn tortilla chips (about 1 oz.)
5 oz. reduced-fat Monterey Jack cheese, shredded
1-⅓ cups drained, rinsed, dried kidney beans
1-⅓ cups drained Mexican-style canned corn kernels
1-⅓ cups chopped fresh cilantro
4 large plum tomatoes, seeded and chopped
5 green onions, chopped
4 generous Tbsp. canned, mild green chilies
12 Tbsp. purchased crushed tomatoes
4 Tbsp. chopped red or green bell peppers

¼ tsp. cayenne pepper
1 onion
Salt to taste

Preparation Instructions:

Preheat oven to 350°F. Arrange tortilla chips closely together on ovenproof plate. Combine ⅓ of cheese, beans, corn, cilantro, tomato, one green onion, and chilies in medium bowl. Mix crushed tomatoes, chopped bell peppers, cayenne, onions, and salt. Add crushed tomato and herb mixture (homemade salsa) and toss to distribute evenly. Spoon vegetable mixture over chips. Sprinkle remaining cheese over. Bake until heated through and cheese on top is melted, about fifteen minutes. Serve immediately. Chopped olives and black beans are also good in this dish.

Herbed Tofu and Portobello Mushrooms with Vegetables

Ingredients for the Mushrooms:

¾ lb. (about 5) plum tomatoes, sliced thick
4 oz. portobello mushrooms, cut into quarter-inch strips
½ yellow bell pepper, chopped
½ yellow onion, halved, with the skin left on
1 shallot with the skin intact
1 head of garlic, the outer skin removed, leaving
    the cloves attached at the root end
2 oz. red pearl onions (available at specialty produce markets)
    or white pearl onions, blanched in boiling water for three
    minutes, drained, and peeled
1 fresh rosemary sprig
1 fresh oregano sprig
1 fresh thyme sprig
3 Tbsp. extra-virgin olive oil
6 oz. tofu
Mixed baby vegetables as an accompaniment
Fresh mint sprigs for garnish

Ingredients for the Mixed Baby Vegetables:

2 oz. baby zucchini and/or baby yellow squash

3 oz. baby carrots, trimmed and peeled
2 oz. thin green beans, trimmed
1 small potato (about ¼ pound)
1 Tbsp. olive oil
½ Tbsp. minced fresh dill and/or mint leaves, or to taste

Preparing the Tofu:

In a large roasting pan, stir together the tomatoes, mushrooms, bell pepper, yellow onion, shallots, garlic, pearl onions, rosemary, oregano, thyme sprig, ⅛ cup of the oil, and salt and pepper to taste. Arrange the tofu, patted dry, on top of the vegetable mixture, drizzle it with the remaining two tablespoons of oil, and season it with salt and pepper. Bake the tofu and the vegetables in the middle of a preheated 300°F oven for fifteen minutes. Reduce the temperature to 200°F and, stirring the vegetables every twenty minutes, bake for twenty minutes more. Transfer the tofu to a platter, spoon the baby vegetables around it, and garnish the tofu with the mint sprigs.

Preparing the Mixed Vegetables:

In a kettle of boiling, salted water, cook separately the zucchini, the pattypan squash, the carrots, and the beans until each vegetable is crisp-tender. Cook the unpeeled potato, and cut into half-inch dice, until it is cooked through. Transfer the cooked vegetables with a spoon to a bowl of ice and cold water to stop the cooking. Drain the vegetables and pat them dry. The vegetables may be prepared up to this point one day in advance and kept covered and chilled. Using moderately high heat, add one tablespoon olive oil in a heavy, nonstick skillet, or use a nonstick lecithin/vegetable spray on a stainless steel pan until it is hot but not smoking. In the pan, sauté the zucchini, the pattypan squash, the carrots, the long beans, and the onions for three minutes, or until they are heated through. Stir in the potato, the herbs, and salt and pepper to taste.

Pasta with Mushrooms, Peppers, and Herbs

Ingredients:

> 2 small red onions, chopped fine
> 2 green bell peppers, chopped fine
> 6 Tbsp. extra-virgin olive oil
> 2 7-oz. jars of roasted red peppers, drained and chopped fine
> 1-½ cup finely sliced mushrooms
> 1 lb. whole-grain spiral pasta
> 2 cups packed mixed basil, mint, and parsley, chopped fine
> Lime wedges
> Romano cheese or non-dairy substitute (available in health-
>   food stores)

Preparation Instructions:

In a heavy, nonstick skillet, or using nonstick lecithin/vegetable spray on a stainless steel pan over moderately low heat, cook onion and green pepper in one tablespoon of oil, stirring until softened, and stir in red peppers and mushrooms. In a kettle of salted, boiling water cook pasta until al dente and drain well. In a bowl toss pasta with pepper mixture, add two tablespoons oil, herbs, and salt and pepper to taste. Serve pasta with lime and Romano.

Tofu Herbal/Vegetable Stew

Ingredients:

> 3 Tbsp. water
> 1 cup zucchini, thinly sliced
> 6 oz. firm tofu
> 1-¼ cups yellow squash, thinly sliced
> ½ cup green bell pepper, cut into 2-inch strips
> ¼ cup celery, cut into 2-inch strips
> ¼ cup onion, chopped
> ½ tsp. caraway seeds
> ⅛ tsp. garlic powder
> 1 medium tomato, cut into eight wedges

Preparation Instructions:
Add first six ingredients to a heavy nonstick skillet or a stainless-steel pan using nonstick lecithin/vegetable spray, over medium heat. Cover and cook four minutes, or until vegetables are just tender. Add remaining ingredients, reduce heat to low, cover, and cook another two minutes.

Buckwheat (Soba) Noodles with Soft Tofu, Garlic, and Herbs
Ingredients:
> 1-½ Tbsp. extra-virgin olive oil and nonstick spray
> ¼ cup thinly sliced garlic
> ¼ cup thinly sliced shallot or scallions
> ¼ cup soft tofu
> ¼ cup warm water
> 2 Tbsp. natural onion soup powder
> 2 Tbsp. rice vinegar
> 1 Tbsp. honey or barley malt syrup (available in health-food stores)
> ½ lb. buckwheat (or whole-wheat) noodles
> ¾ small onion, sliced thin
> 1 small red bell pepper, cut into thin strips
> ½ pint vine-ripened cherry tomatoes, quartered
> ⅛ cup thinly sliced fresh basil leaves
> ⅛ cup chopped fresh coriander

Preparation Instructions:
In an eight- or nine-inch skillet, heat nonstick spray over moderate heat until hot but not smoking. Sauté shallot or scallions, stirring, for one to two minutes. Sauté garlic in the same manner.

In a large bowl soak noodles in cold water to cover fifteen minutes. Drain noodles, and in a kettle of boiling water cook until just tender, one to two minutes. In a colander drain noodles and rinse under cold water. Drain noodles well. In a large skillet sauté onion and bell pepper in two tablespoons oil over moderate heat, stirring until softened, and add tomatoes, tofu, noodles, and onion powder. Cook mixture, stirring, until heated through. Add basil and coriander, garlic, and shallots, and toss noodles well.

Mock "Hot Lasagna"

Ingredients:

3 medium potatoes
3 cups crushed tomatoes
¼ Tbsp. Italian seasoning
A pinch cayenne pepper
16 oz. firm tofu
⅓ cup fresh lime or lemon juice
2 cloves fresh, minced garlic
3 tsp. dried basil
3 tsp. dried oregano
Salt or soy sauce to taste
6 cups fresh, shredded collard greens
¾ cup shredded soy cheese

Preparation Instructions:

Boil, bake, or microwave potatoes and cool for at least thirty minutes. Meanwhile, mix crushed tomatoes with Italian seasoning and cayenne. With a fork, whip the tofu, lime or lemon juice, oregano, basil, and garlic until smooth. To create lasagna, cover the bottom of a 9 x 13-inch steel or glass baking pan with about ⅓ of the crushed tomato, salt, and herb mixture. Cover this with two potatoes, thinly sliced. Now layer one after the other with half of the tofu mixture, the fresh collard greens, and a third of the tomato sauce. Complete the process with another layer of potatoes, and the remaining tofu mixture and crushed tomato and herb mixture sauce. Cover the entire dish with soy cheese. Bake at 375°F for forty-five minutes. Let stand for fifteen minutes. This dish is delicious served with whole-grain sourdough bread and fresh fruit.

Scalloped Potatoes with Low-Fat Cottage Cheese and Herbs de Provence

Herbes de Provence is an herbal blend that consists of a blend of dried herbs, usually basil, thyme, rosemary, and oregano, and occasionally lavender.

Ingredients:

¾ cup vegetable broth

¼ cup minced shallots

½ Tbsp. minced garlic

2 tsp. Herbs de Provence

¼ tsp. sea salt

⅛ tsp. of arrowroot starch

5 oz. 1 percent cottage cheese

2 lbs. russet potatoes, peeled and thinly sliced

Preparation Instructions:

Preheat your oven to 400°F. Spray nonstick vegetable spray on a 13 x 9 x 2-inch glass baking dish. Combine the first five ingredients in a large pot. Simmer over medium-high heat. Add half of the cheese and mix in. Chill remaining cheese. Add potatoes to pot, and bring to simmer. Mix arrowroot starch with water and stir until smooth. Add the arrowroot to the mixture. Transfer potato mixture to prepared dish, spreading evenly. Cover with foil; bake fifteen minutes. Uncover and bake until potatoes are very tender and liquid bubbles thickly, about fifty minutes. Dot potatoes with remaining cheese. Bake until cheese softens, about five minutes. Allow it to cool fifteen minutes before serving.

Broccoli and Garlic-Stuffed Potatoes

Ingredients:

4 baking potatoes, scrubbed

½ cup low-fat cottage cheese

4 clove chopped garlic

8 Tbsp. plus 2 tsp. prepared broccoli

4 Tbsp. plus 1 tsp. extra-virgin olive oil

4 Tbsp. plus 1 tsp. chives

4 Tbsp. low-fat yogurt

Preparation Instructions:
Preheat oven to 400°F. Pierce potatoes several times with a fork. Bake about one hour, or until crisp outside and cooked through. Transfer to a baking sheet and cool five minutes. Lightly steam broccoli. Cut off the top third of the potatoes. Scoop out potato from bottoms into a bowl, leaving a quarter-inch thick shell. Scoop potato from tops and add to same bowl. Discard tops. Mash potato with half the cottage cheese, half the chopped garlic, and olive oil. Season with salt and pepper to taste. Spoon into potato shells, dividing equally. Place potatoes in baking pan and bake about twenty minutes, or until heated through and golden brown. Mix remaining cottage cheese and garlic. Spoon yogurt topping on the potato and sprinkle with chives.

Herbed Tofu Pilaf
Ingredients:
15 oz. Vegebase or vegetable powder mixed in distilled water
1-¼ cup cracked wheat
¾ tsp. basil, crumbled
½ tsp. mint flakes
¾ tsp. grated, organically grown lemon rind
¾ cup whole, natural (unblanched) almonds
1-½ Tbsp. almond or olive oil
¾ cup sliced green onion
½ cup seedless raisins or currants
3 Tbsp. chopped parsley
1-½ Tbsp. lemon juice
1-¼ cup diced Tofu

Preparation Instructions:
Combine twelve ounces of Vegebase and water with cracked wheat, basil, mint flakes, and lemon rind, and heat to boiling. Cover, turn heat low, and cook fifteen minutes. Meanwhile, chop almonds. When cracked wheat is cooked, add almonds, onion, raisins (currants), parsley, and lemon juice; toss lightly to mix. Add tofu and heat a minute longer.

Herbed Egg Salad Sandwiches
Ingredients:
> 1 lb. firm tofu, mashed
> 4 Tbsp. eggless mayonnaise
>   (available at specialty- and natural-food stores)
> 4 Tbsp. yogurt
> 4 Tbsp. minced fresh parsley, chives, and/or tarragon
> 2 scallions, minced
> 4 tsp. fresh lemon juice, or to taste
> 4 tsp. Dijon mustard
> A pinch of lemon juice
> 8 slices whole-grain sourdough bread

Preparation Instructions:
In a bowl stir together all ingredients (except bread) with salt and pepper to taste until combined well.

Herbed Tricolor Pasta Salad
Ingredients:
> ½ cup plain yogurt
> ¼ cup eggless mayonnaise (available in health-food stores)
> ½ Tbsp. white wine vinegar, or to taste
> ¼ cup minced fresh parsley leaves
> Small red onion, quartered and sliced thin
> ¼ cup finely chopped assorted fresh herbs such as basil,
>   dill, and chives
> ½ lb. tricolor pasta such as penne or fusilli

Preparing Dressing:
In a large bowl whisk together yogurt, eggless mayonnaise, vinegar, parsley, onion, and herbs. In a kettle of boiling, salted, bottled water cook pasta until tender, about twelve minutes. In a large colander drain pasta and rinse well under cold water. Allow the pasta to drain well and toss with dressing and salt and pepper to taste. Pasta salad may be made four hours ahead and chilled, covered. If pasta absorbs dressing while standing, toss with about one tablespoon warm water.

Herbed Dessert Recipes

One of the most difficult elements in any weight-management program is fulfilling a desire for sweets without eating foods that are high in refined sugar, fat, and artificial ingredients. For instance, the characteristic colors we associate with different flavors of puddings, gelatin desserts, frozen desserts, and prepared mixes are provided almost entirely by synthetic coloring agents. More than 90 percent are synthetically produced, while the others are derived from plants. These natural dessert recipes were created so that they are rich in flavor and texture, and low in fat and calories.

Most of the dessert recipes listed here are moderate to high on the glycemic index. If used in moderation, these banana recipes can create a great dessert or snack food, and are a wonderful addition to a weight-management program because they are rich in texture, sweet to the taste, and highly versatile. A nutrition powerhouse, bananas are rich in potassium, magnesium, and vitamin B6. Research indicates that potassium may have a greater influence on lowering high blood pressure than even reducing sodium levels. Magnesium may have a similar influence on blood pressure and may play an important role in reducing the risk of heart disease. The fact that a banana has a higher caloric content than an equal amount of most other fruits is not problematic. Bananas are sweeter and more filling than many other fruits, and can be used as a substitute for other foods that might have higher levels of fat calories. It is best to eat yellow bananas (Cavendish Variety) when they start to form brown spots. This is when they are at their best, sweet and rich. There are also small, plump red bananas that are rich in texture and intense in their sweet flavor. Plantains are a type of starchy banana that are used in many different cuisines and are often prepared in a similar manner as a starchy root vegetable. Yellow and red bananas make a great dessert. Unripe bananas should never be refrigerated since they will never ripen, but overripe bananas can be frozen and used as an ice-cream replacement. The best way to use them is to peel them and wrap them in plastic or wax paper before freezing. They may turn dark brown or black but this will do them no harm.

Use bananas as low-calorie desserts or snacks:

- Place a frozen banana in a food processor and serve with low-fat carob or other dessert topping from a health-food store.
- Make a frozen banana pop. Place a pop stick into a peeled banana, dip it in any type of fruit juice, and roll it in low-fat granola. Now freeze. When they are firm, they are ready to eat.
- Mash half a banana and mix it with a teaspoon of any nut butter. Spread this on a rice cake.

Banana Pudding

Ingredients:

10 oz. soft, silken tofu
2 bananas, ripe
Maple syrup to taste

Preparation Instructions:

Blend banana with tofu and maple syrup until smooth. Pour into serving cups. Chill for one to two hours. Before serving, top with fresh sliced fruit such as bananas or blueberries.

Fruit Celebration

Ingredients:

2 cups non-fat vanilla yogurt (or plain yogurt with natural vanilla extract added)
¼ lb. fresh, chopped pineapple chunks
1 large plum, thinly sliced
1 ripe, firm banana, peeled and thinly sliced
1 large ripe mango, peeled and thinly sliced
2 Tbsp. flaxseed

Preparation Instructions:

Combine all ingredients in a mixing bowl and toss. Chill before serving.

Broiled Cinnamon Maple Plantains
Ingredients:

> 4 plantains, cut in half lengthwise
> ¼ cup natural maple syrup
> Nonstick lecithin/vegetable spray
> 2 cups non-fat vanilla yogurt (or plain yogurt with natural
>   vanilla extract added)
> ½ cup finely chopped pineapple

Preparation Instructions:
Turn on broiler. Arrange bananas in a shallow baking dish. Drizzle with maple syrup. Place under broiler two to three minutes or until honey is bubbly and bananas are glazed. Serve bananas with a dollop of yogurt and chopped pineapple.

Herbed Banana Date Nut Salad
Ingredients:

> 2 bananas, peeled and cut into half-inch slices
> 8 dates, pitted and chopped
> ¼ cup chopped pecans
> 1 tsp. lemon juice
> A pinch of nutmeg to taste

Preparation Instructions:
Combine bananas, dates, and pecans in a mixing bowl. Sprinkle with lemon juice and toss. Serve in a dessert dish.

Tofu Blueberry Pudding
Ingredients:

> 1-½ lbs. medium tofu
> 1-½ tsp. alcohol-free vanilla extract
> 2 tsp. lemon juice
> 10 oz. blueberries
> 1 ripe banana, mashed
> ½ cup honey

Preparation Instructions:

Thaw and drain raspberries. Blend all ingredients until creamy. Chill and serve.

Herbal Tea Recipes

Purification Tea

Combine:

> 1 Tbsp. each of mullein and spearmint
>
> ¾ Tbsp. each of rosehips, organic orange peel, a pinch of
> goldenseal

Basic Cleansing Juice

Combine:

> 7 oz. carrot juice
>
> 6 oz. cucumber juice
>
> 2 oz. parsley juice
>
> 1 oz. beet juice

Fresh Vegetables

Beets, Boston lettuce, broccoli, cauliflower, celery, corn on the cob, cucumbers, green peas, green peppers, kale, mushrooms, radishes, Romaine lettuce, scallions, shallots, squash, tomatoes, watercress, white potatoes

Fresh Fruit, Nuts, and Seeds

Apples, bananas, grapes, lemons, peaches (and/or nectarines), pineapple, almonds (slivered), breadcrumbs (whole wheat), bulgur, cereal (puffed brown rice or millet), cereal (granola), canola oil, filberts, soy, flour (whole wheat or other grain), fruit juice, frozen concentrate, herbal tea or coffee substitute

Herbs and Spices

Basil (fresh), bay leaves, cayenne, chili powder, chives (dried), cinnamon, coriander, curry powder, cumin, garlic (fresh), mint leaves (dried), mustard powder (dried), onion powder, oregano (dried), parsley (fresh), peppercorns (black and white), rosemary (fresh or dried), sage (fresh or dried), honey, kelp, lemon rind, milk (low-fat), millet, oatmeal, olive oil (extra virgin), orange juice, pasta (whole wheat), peppers (hot), pine nuts (unroasted), raisins (or dried currants), raspberries (frozen), rice (brown), rice milk, sea salt, sesame seeds (raw), soy grits or granules, soy milk, soy sauce (low sodium), sunflower seeds (raw), tempeh, tofu (medium and firm), tomato paste, tomatoes (crushed, canned), TVP (textured vegetable protein), vanilla extract (alcohol-free), vegebase brand powder, vinegar, apple cider, distilled water, yogurt (non-fat, plain or flavored)

Bibliography

Dartnell Corporation, *Sad News for Dieters*, Working Together Bulletin, 1986.

Gilliard, Judy. *Cooking with Herbs & Spices*. Adams Media Corporation: Massachusetts, 1999.

Hirsch, Alan R. *Scentsational Weight Loss*. Fireside Books: New York, 1998.

Jantz, Gregory L. *The Spiritual Path to Weight Loss*. Publications International, LTD: Lincolnwood, 1998.

Journal of Chinese Medicine. www.jcm.co.uk/news. 14 May 2002.

La Ferla, Ruth. "Beauty Goes Fruity." *New York Times* 28 Jan. 2001.

Levine, Jeff. "Doctors Say Exercise, Tomatoes Can Cut Cancer." www.cnn.com/health/9703/24/nfm/cancer.exercise. 14 May 2002.

Lust, John. *The Herb Book*. Bantam Dell: New York, 1974.

Mowrey, Daniel B. *Fat Management! The Thermogenic Factor*. Victory: Lehi, 1994.

Noell, M.D., Courtney. eMedicine Journal. Vol.2, No.10. www.emedicine.com/ent/topic333. 14 May 2002.

Pritikin, Robert. *The Pritikin Weight Loss Breakthrough*. Dutton: New York, 1998.

"Research Lifts Blame From Many of the Obese," *New York Times* 24 March 1987.

Rinzler, Carol Ann. *The Complete Book of Herbs, Spices, and Condiments*. Facts on File, Inc.: New York, 1990.

Rose, Jeanne. *Jeanne Rose's Herbal Guide to Food*. North Atlantic Books: Berkeley, 1989.

Smith, Susan Male and Densie Webb. *Fat Fighting Food*. Publications International, LTD.: Lincolnwood, 1997.

Tufts University Diet & Nutrition Newsletter 3.1 (March 1985): 5.

Walker, N.W., *Raw Vegetable Juices*, Berkley Publishers: New York, 1991.

Weiss, Linda. *Kitchen Magic by Linda Weiss*. Keats Publishing, Inc.: New Canaan, 1994.

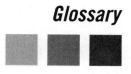

Acidophilus: One of a number of healthy bacteria that are helpful in both improving digestion and in body detoxification. These bacteria are the same as those used to culture various sour food products, including yogurt.

Alpha Lipoic Acid: A co-factor for a key enzyme (alpha keto acid dehydrogeneses) involved in generating energy from food and oxygen in mitochondria. Known as a "Universal antioxidant," Alpha lipoic acid is found in virtually every cell of the body, and it counteracts excessive free radical activity via several mechanisms in cell membranes as well as inside cells.

Antioxidant: Chemical factors, often nutrients that can reduce the negative effects of oxidation, specifically the formation of free radicals, by stopping or reducing oxidation in those places in the body where it may be harmful.

Aromatherapy: Therapeutic applications of essential oils.

Ayurveda: A traditional East Indian medical and healing system developed from ancient texts known as the Vedas. Many of the techniques used in Ayurveda involve herbs.

Bach Remedies: Homeopathically prepared flower essences that influence balance and reduce emotional stress and trauma.

Calorie: A measure of heat in the body.

Carrier or Base Oil: An oil, usually derived from seeds or other plant substances that have little or no aroma of their own and are used in preparing aromatherapy massage oils.

Cayenne (Capsicum frutescens): This red powder is used as a culinary spice as well as for its healing properties. It stimulates the production of ATP (fuel), thus increasing thermogenesis and stimulating the BAT cells so more calories are burned.

Complex Carbohydrates: An essential nutrient necessary for the functioning of your brain and nervous system. They also supply energy for digestion and muscular exertion, and are necessary for proper absorption of other foods. Carbohydrates provide glucose for nerve tissues and provide a primary source of energy.

Cuwijia: This herb is used in Chinese medicine to bolster fatigue and enhance immune activity, but Chinese researchers also note that the herb increases the burning of fat during strenuous exercise.

Detoxification: The process by which the body neutralizes the waste products of metabolism, purifies the blood, and cleanses the tissues in the body. Herbs and spices, especially in combination with juicing, are particularly effective in helping a person in detoxification.

Dioscorides: A first-century Greek physician and botanist. For fifteen hundred years his reference work *De Materia Medica* was the standard work on botany and the therapeutic use of plants.

Ephedra: An ingredient used in many commercial herbal products. Also known as ma huang, it is often combined with caffeine. Ephedra is a powerful stimulant and thermogenic compound with the potential to affect the nervous system and heart. When used properly it is generally safe, but it can be overused, which can lead to health problems, high blood pressure, heart rate irregularities, insomnia, nervousness, tremors, headaches, and even seizures, heart attacks, and strokes.

Essential Oil: Aromatic oil derived from plants. They have a strong aroma and were the original basis for most perfumes. Essential oils are valuable tools for healing the body and mind.

Fat: An essential nutrient that includes complex combinations of what we call lipids, fatty substances that include fat-soluble vitamins, tocopherols, triglycerides, sterols, and phospholipids.

These supply the essential fatty acids needed for innumerable glandular and metabolic processes. They also are a primary source of energy for the body

Fen-phen: The anti-obesity prescription drugs dexfenfluramine (brand name Redux) and fenfluramine (brand name Pondimin). They were withdrawn from the marketplace because of complaints concerning their safety.

Fiber: The portion of a plant that has not been digested by enzymes in the intestinal tract.

Flax: A seed that is high in essential fatty acids. These work with the physiologic and metabolic processes in the body. Flaxseed oil also helps to regulate blood sugar and insulin levels.

Garcinia Cambogia: Derived from a dried jungle berry native to India, this is among the most effective and balanced of herbs that promote weight loss. Rich in hydroxycitric acid (also called hydrocitrate or HCA).

Ginger: A perennial, ginger grows in Southern Asia, Mexico, Jamaica, and other countries. Ginger increases blood circulation, aids in the metabolism of dietary nutrients, and plays an important role in Ayurvedic treatments as well. Ginger oil is very popular as a healing tool in aromatherapy.

Glucomannan: Glucomannan is a calorie-free, high-fiber herb, which is obtained from the root of the Amorphophallus Konjac plant.

Glycemic Index: A scale of how foods are metabolized, the Glycemic Index measures the effect an individual food has on blood sugar (glucose) levels.

Green Tea: A beverage noted for its antioxidant properties.

Guggulipid: Guggul is a gummy resin that oozes from a tree (Commiphora mukul) that grows in India. The plant contains compounds called guggulsterones that have been proven to regulate metabolism. Guggulipid also stimulates the BAT cells, thus increasing thermogenesis and burning stored fat.

Gymnema Sylvestre: This herb, also know as Gurmar, has been used in Ayurvedic medicine for more than two thousand years to control problems in carbohydrate metabolism, particularly concerning obesity and diabetes. Another valuable aspect of this herb is that it appears to reduce cravings for sweet foods through its influence on the taste receptors.

HGH (Human Growth Hormone): A hormone that helps people burn fat and build muscle. Research has indicated that HGH, which is present at high levels in children to meet the needs of rapidly growing bodies, is released at a slower pace as a person reaches thirty years old, and virtually stops after thirty. Nutritional scientists also believe that this hormone is dormant in individuals who are plagued by obesity, whatever their age.

Lacto Vegetarian: *see* Vegetarian

Lacto-ovo Vegetarian: *see* Vegetarian

Licorice: A perennial plant native to Southern Europe and Asia. This ancient Egyptian cure-all is also called *liquorice,* meaning "the sweet root." Its roots and rhizomes are prized both medicinally and for their sweet flavoring.

Linoleic Acid : One of the two essential fatty acids.

Lipoprotein Lipase (LPL): An enzyme factor that may influence obesity. LPL helps the body store excess calories in fat cells. The enzyme is manufactured in fat cells and is transported to the capillaries, where it breaks dietary fat into tiny particles that penetrate the membranes of these fat cells.

Lycopene: This natural antioxidant found exclusively in tomatoes is getting much attention in the press as a cancer fighter.

Ma Huang: An herb found in many commercial weight-loss formulas. Its active ingredient, ephedrine, is the most effective thermogenic. The consumption of ma huang can result in unwanted side effects for some people.

Milk Thistle: A member of the sunflower family, more than three hundred scientific studies attest to the benefits of this herb, particularly in detoxification of the liver.

Mineral: A non-caloric essential nutrient used in the development of blood, nerves, bones, teeth, and other tissues; restoration of an acid-based balance; and maintenance of proper bodily processes.

Mustard Seeds: Used since ancient times as a medicine, mustard seeds possess a thermogenic quality.

Myrrh: A smokey herb derived from a tree resin that has a centering quality that assists in emotional stabilization, visualization, and meditation. It is one of the oldest-known aromatic materials, and is associated with gifts brought to the infant Jesus.

Neurotransmitters: Multifunctional chemicals in the brain that allow nerve impulses to move from neuron to neuron. In detecting and reacting to odors, the neurons move from the olfactory bulb through the limbic lobe. Neurotransmitters are also responsible for emotional well-being and the regulation of moods.

Obesity: When a person takes in more calories than he or she uses, and stores the excess calories are as fat. As a rule of thumb, if you are carrying 25 percent or more of your body weight in fat, you are obese.

Pectin: A water-soluble fiber that is found in plant cells.

Peppermint: One of the most popular herbs in the world, as well as one of the most important oils.

Pheromones: Odorous substances that abound in the human and animal world. It is believed that these scents were responsible for man's early survival and, through the years, have been replaced with our reliance on vision.

Protein: An essential nutrient that is needed by the body to restore and renew body tissue and cells, ensure proper distribution of fluids throughout the body, and maintain bodily functions and create antibodies for the immune system.

Sea Vegetables: Herbs and plants harvested from the oceans. They are high in minerals and are popular in many weight-management programs because they have been found by some to stimulate a sluggish thyroid and reduce the constipation that some people experience on high-protein, low-carbohydrate diets.

Shaman: A healer, found in many cultures, who simultaneously serves as a religious leader, spiritual teacher, and medicine man.

Spirulina: Spirulina is a type of micro algae. Micro algaes are aquatic plants that have no roots, leaves, seeds, or flowers. Many varieties are used in commercial weight-loss formulas because they are a rich source of nutrients that can easily absorbed by the body.

St. John's Wort: This yellow-flowered plant is found in many herbal fen-phen products. Recent studies indicate that it is a mood elevator and may curb overeating associated with depression.

Tempeh: Tempeh is a fermented soy product that is a staple food in Indonesia. Tempeh serves as a meat substitute and can be baked, steamed, boiled, or grilled.

Thermogenesis: The body's tendency to burn brown fat by increasing the production of heat-energy, which burns calories.

Tissue Salts: Tissue Salts, also known as cell salts, are vibrationally based, homeopathically prepared remedies.

Tofu: Tofu, a bland, custard-like food made from soybeans, is the most popular and versatile of all of the soyfoods. A complete protein containing all eight essential amino acids, tofu is also rich in vitamins, minerals, fatty acids, and other nutrients.

Turmeric: An herb noted for its antioxidant properties.

Vitamin: A non-caloric essential nutrient used to optimize the function of nutrients from food and other vitamins and facilitate the maintenance of bodily processes.

Vegan: *see* Vegetarian

Vegetarian: An approach to nutrition that eliminates the use of meat, fish, or poultry. Lacto vegetarians use milk products but do not include eggs in their diet. Lacto-ovo vegetarians use eggs. Vegans avoid all products derived from animals.

Yerba Maté: This herb, commonly called maté, is an evergreen member of the holly family. Yerbe Maté contains mateins, a substance similar to caffeine, which energizes but does not jangle and overstimulate the nervous system, and seems to lack most of the negative side effects associated with caffeine.

Visualization: A stress-management and general-healing technique that involves using mental images to reduce stress and influence behavior.

Index

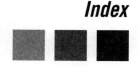

About the Author

Lewis Harrison is the author of six books on human potential including *Hands-on Healing*. The former host of a talk radio show in NYC, he is now the director of The Academy of Natural Healing and has been an instructor at the prestigious New York Botanical Gardens. He presently speaks on stress management to corporate and college audiences and through his "Master Your Metabolism" seminars. He may be contacted at www.chihealer.com.